Natural R

Ultimate Guide on H
Improved Health - Eliminate Fatigue and Stop
Procrastination (Use Natural Cures To Beat
Anxiety, Panic Attacks, Inflammation, Colds And
Flu)

Brad J Johnson

Published By **Zoe Lawson**

Brad J Johnson

All Rights Reserved

Natural Remedies: Ultimate Guide on Herbal Remedies For Improved Health - Eliminate Fatigue and Stop Procrastination (Use Natural Cures To Beat Anxiety, Panic Attacks, Inflammation, Colds And Flu)

ISBN 978-1-77485-511-9

Legal & Disclaimer

The information contained in this ebook is not designed to replace or take the place of any form of medicine or professional medical advice. The information in this ebook has been provided for educational & entertainment purposes only.

The information contained in this book has been compiled from sources deemed reliable, and it is accurate to the best of the Author's knowledge; however, the Author cannot guarantee its accuracy and validity and cannot be held liable for any errors or omissions. Changes are periodically made to this book. You must consult your doctor or get professional medical advice before using any of the suggested remedies, techniques, or information in this book.

Upon using the information contained in this book, you agree to hold harmless the Author from and against any damages, costs, and expenses, including any legal fees potentially resulting from the application of any of the information provided by this guide. This disclaimer applies to any damages or injury caused by the use and application, whether directly or indirectly, of any advice or information presented, whether for breach of contract, tort, negligence, personal injury, criminal intent, or under any other cause of action.

You agree to accept all risks of using the information presented inside this book. You need to consult a professional medical practitioner in order to ensure you are both able and healthy enough to participate in this program.

Table of Contents

Chapter 1: General Information.................................. 1

Chapter 2: How Does It Work 3

Chapter 3: Different Herbs And Their Applications....10

Chapter 4: Natural Remedies To Overcome Anxiety..39

Chapter 5: Common Herbal Medicines 43

Chapter 6: Natural Remedies For Mild Infections......57

Chapter 7: Herbs To Treat Common Ailments...........63

Chapter 8: Herbal Remedies For Children 88

Chapter 9: Herbals To Treat Skin Problems 102

Chapter 10: Home Remedies For Ligament, Joint, Tendons And Joint Conditions 109

Chapter 11: Herbs For Curing Pain And Inflammation 115

Chapter 12: Facial Scrubs.......................................118

Chapter 13: Headache And Fever Solutions 127

Chapter 14: Superior Beverages Options 131

Chapter 15: Utilizing Natural Supplements To Cure Insomnia 136

Chapter 16: Medicinal Herbs And Essential Oils 140

Chapter 17: Green And Red Tea...............................147

Chapter 18: Supplements And Herbs For Hypertension 163

Chapter 19: Corns And Chilblains............................169

Chapter 20: Using Essential Oils For Natural Cures..178

Chapter 21: Natural Remedies For Hair Loss 181

Chapter 1: General Information

Before we begin in the kitchen with recipes, and suggestions, it is appropriate to provide some basic guidelines about the idea of herbalism and what exactly the characteristics of our Earth Earth can aid in fighting illnesses and improve our overall health.

Herbalism, often known as herbology and herbology, can be described as a strategy to treat diseases that date to long before Christ. It is the practice of using various plants and combinations of natural substances which can alter the chemistry of our bodies positively. It is, in actual the method used by doctors to treat illnesses for the majority of the history of humanity. This conventional medicine has only recently made a return in recent times.

Herbalism is seen by modern medicine to be in the area in the category of "alternative medicine" because it is believed to be a form of medicine that is not supported by scientific research. This is a somewhat biased opinion, since an enormous portion of modern pharmaceutical production is based on herbal base. A variety of compounds that are derived from plants are used in the production of phototherapy and drugs, since they are directly connected to the human body as well as its roles.

It's true, bee and fungal products are an integral part of herbalism, and as you'll discover in this book, they play an important place in many home remedies and recipes.

Chapter 2: How Does It Work

There is no doubt that a lot of people are skeptical about the ability of herbal remedies to treat ailments and their effectiveness in modern times. But, what doctors from the past were able to do was to study the effects of herbs in the body of a person. Yes, there were some undesirable situations, but it was a matter of discovering what was beneficial and which are not. At the time, they didn't have the latest technology, which is the reason they had to test in this manner.

As time passed it became clear that there was enough information to turn it into an actual science. At the time, the herbal treatments worked perfectly as evidenced by the evidence of history that show those who could afford to buy the services of these doctors usually lived long lives according to the standards of their time. Today , we're fortunate enough to have this knowledge available in books and on the internet. In addition, we have access to the majority of resources in addition to specific instructions on what to do with them.

As we have mentioned in the beginning of the chapter, a significant component of modern-day drugstore medicine is in fact based on a natural base. There are many active ingredients extracted from plants. Sometimes, the most significant difference between pharmaceuticals and herbal blends is that the former are created in a laboratory and are formulated like pills. According to estimates, about eighty percent of the population worldwide uses plants as part of their health. It is estimated that the United States alone has more than one thousand and five hundred botanicals that are offered as supplements. All over the world, people are taking advantage of various plants to treat common ailments and ailments. In this book, we are trying to teach you how to increase your knowledge about the topic and treat yourself with respect, and without resorting to chemicals that cause a reaction.

The benefits of Taheebo Tea

The many advantages that come from Taheebo

Tea that are taken benefit of are directly attributed to its fundamental characteristics. To comprehend how Taheebo Tea is beneficial to the body, it's first essential to understand what the benefits of its properties are.

As mentioned earlier in the previous paragraph, Taheebo Tea as well as the Pau d'Arco generally is antifungal and antibacterial in nature. Due to these properties it's highly effective in treating many other diseases that are common. It is active against fungi, bacterial and yeast growth. They include Staphylococcus dysentery, pneumonia, Bucella, tuberculosis, Aspergillus and the most common reason for stomach ulcers: Helicobacter Pylori. It also has been proven to have a potent in vitro action against viruses, including the vesicular stomatitis virus, polio Herpes I and II and influenza. Furthermore, it is proven to be anti-parasitic for tropical diseases like the schistosoma virus, malaria, and typanosoma. It was also effective as an expectorant which enabled it to increase coughing. This helped the lungs expel mucus, a substance that is deeply embedded in contaminates being one of them.

The health benefits derived from a variety of

5

chemicals that are present within the tree's bark. These chemicals include lapachone isolapachone and lapachol. The majority of medical professionals believe that tannins are an important natural remedy and that these chemical compounds are secondarily related to tannins. Taheebo tea is antifungal and antibacterial, as well as helping fight tumors, it's an effective treatment for many illnesses. Additionally, it stimulates an increase in the number of red blood cells which makes it a valuable component for treating leukemia and other blood-related ailments.

One of the main reasons it is one of the most effective methods to fight diseases in the modern world is that the many side negative effects that can be seen when using western medicines, including hair loss, pain , and immune dysfunction are not present with taheebo. This is why it is possible to make use of tea taheebo in conjunction with other medical treatments. Additionally, research has shown that patients undergoing chemotherapy saw a reduction in side effects as the efficacy of chemotherapy improved. Thus, it has proved to be one of the most promising therapies as far as the tumor and cancer are involved because of the absence of numerous adverse consequences.

The advantages of taheebo don't stop there because it is also utilized to treat minor differences. It is utilized as a poultice to treat eye inflammation, or as a wash for yeast infections, and even helps in healing sores and open wounds. Therefore it is not just flexible for us, but it's also affordable, which is a testament to its position as the central point of rituals of healing for the tribal people for generations.

Additionally, it's employed in the treatment of constipation. It also aids in strengthening the immune system, and fight chronic illnesses. It also aids with replenishing essential elements which makes it healthier as well as improving appetite. It is also used as a poultice for treating many skin ailments like the skin cancers, eczema fungal infections , and psoriasis. Experts also suggest it aids in fighting viral infections like AIDS and AIDS, too. It can also be used to treat chronic inflammation, such as the hardening of arteries as well as arthritis.

It is considered to be one of the most original plant extracts, taheebo is utilized to treat daily problems like increasing hair growth and diminishing age spots. It is not just linked to age spots, as it also blocks free radicals, it's also an anti-aging herbal remedy. It also lessens the dependence on insulin among some insulin-dependent diabetics. Due to its high iron content it can enhance the absorption of other nutrients too.

One of the greatest benefits of taheebo is that it can help with cases which were thought to be insurmountable using allopathic medicines. It reenergizes the body since it makes new normal cells, and also increases the resistance to illness. Taheebo can stimulate the digestive tract via the rectum, and then back into the gall bladder as well as the liver and sweat glands, which act as relief valves for the lungs stomach, and heart. Therefore, it is not just helpful in keeping the glands in good working order and eliminates issues that originate from stomach acid, but it can also trigger warning signs for the body when adrenal glands are stressed.

It is known for its healing properties and is believed to boost immune system cells called macrophanges to take action. As tests were carried out, it was successful in eliminating lung cancer cells as well as liver cancer cells growing in test tubes . It also reduced lung cancer in mice following surgery which eliminated the tumor.

Taheebo tea also has an abundance of iron that is easily absorbed. It slowly eliminates pain, and it can increase the quantity of blood red cells. This helps the body to be in an armed position, which helps to protect itself from illnesses.

Chapter 3: Different Herbs And Their Applications

There are hundreds of thousands of plants utilized to treat various types of illnesses. Choosing which one to utilize is a difficult task. This chapter will be more in-depth on the different medicinal herbs and their use to treat various ailments.

Cayenne Pepper

Cayenne Pepper is a type of chili which belongs to the Family Solanaceae. Cayenne pepper is a source of the compound capsaicin which helps to boost metabolism. It is a great food to improve the health of those suffering from heart issues, migraine or headache. The consumption of cayenne pepper may also reduce inflammation in the body and reduce pain and discomfort in the body. It can also be put into a topical remedy such as an ointment that is applied on the skin for treatment of the pain and arthritis that is localized in the body. Additionally, it has antibacterial qualities which can be utilized to treat the symptoms of psoriasis.

Eucalyptus

Eucalyptus is the flowering plant well-known for its fragrant leaves. The leaves are frequently utilized for aromatherapy. The leaves are a source of 70 percent cineole. Additionally, it contains chemical compounds like pinenes, aromadendrene, cuminaldehyde as well as sesquiterpene alcohols. These chemicals open the lungs and clear the nasal passageway of any obstruction. This is what makes Eucalyptus an effective treatment for fighting influenza and colds.

Eucalyptus oil is used for a variety of purposes and in addition to treating flu and colds it is also utilized to treat arthritis, burns and bronchitis, as well as wounds, as well as sore throat. Additionally, eucalyptus oil can be utilized as a repellent for insects and is believed for its effectiveness in eliminating lice.

Eucalyptus is a plant that can be consumed as tea, in addition to steam inhalations. If you drink it in the form of tea Eucalyptus tea can be used to cool the body and soothes the nasal passages, thus improving the overall health of those who is suffering from flu or cold.

Ginger

Ginger is a special root (rhizome) that is considered as a major commercial crop. Ginger is a rich source of different compounds that comprise bisabolene, oleoresin gingerols and zingerone as well as Zingiberone and shoagaols. It also has Vitamins A as well as B, in addition to other minerals. Ginger is a common herb that is not only used in cooking , but it can also be utilized to treat various ailments such as dysmenorrhea, indigestion asthma, flu, arthritis and nausea.

Ginger is also utilized in aromatherapy. It is also recognized as being efficient in improving cardiovascular health since it is thought as an anti-inflammatory and blood thinner. It also helps lower cholesterol levels in the body.

Ginger is a great ingredient to mix with other herbs and enhances the effectiveness and potency of infusions made from herbs. It is generally made into tea. The strong smell and spicy taste make the ginger tea very effective to clear nasal passages in those suffering from flu and colds. To enhance the effectiveness of the ginger tea, sipping it with honey and lemon can provide many benefits, including easing those symptoms associated with motion sickness as well as nausea following surgery.

Rosemary

The herb of rosemary is versatile that can be used to enhance the taste of various food items. In addition to adding flavor to fooditems, the flowers, leaves as well as the stems are additionally used to treat various diseases like arthritis, bronchitis hypertension, scabies, and cuts. Rosemary is also believed to boost circulation, cardiovascular health and as well as reduce the risk of developing diabetes. In addition, the smell of rosemary has been proven to enhance memory and alleviate people suffering from stress and anxiety.

The rosemary plant contains compounds like the limonene compound, camphor as well as cineole, borneol, and camphene. It also has flavonoids, phenolic acid, diterpenes, rosmarinic acid and triterpenes. It is processed often in order to obtain its oil. The consumption of essential oils from rosemary could help in preventing rheumatic ailments as well as ease the symptoms associated with circulatory issues. It is also used as an ointment to apply to areas of the hair and skin to improve the health of the body's organs. Apart from extracting the vital oil from rosemary, it can be utilized in cooking to increase the nutritional content of food you consume.

Turmeric

Turmeric is among the most potent herbs and is well-known for its anti-cancer properties. The component used in turmeric is called the Rhizome. Rhizomes contain volatile oils like curcumen, terpene and curcumen that are believed to have anti-cancer properties of rhizomes. Additionally, the rhizome has high levels of Potassium and Vitamin C.

Numerous studies verify the anti-inflammatory qualities of turmeric. It is a rich source of compounds that can help reduce the inflammation that occurs inside and outside of the body. It is able to inhibit the production of prostaglandin, a hormone which is responsible for inflammation. Because of this, turmeric is not just an option for treating cancer but also cataracts and Alzheimer's disease. Furthermore, turmeric could be utilized to treat rheumatoid arthritis. Turmeric is typically consumed in the form of a powder or as a supplementation. It also can be used in conjunction together with pepper and ginger to help activate the effects of turmeric. A tea infusion that is made of turmeric also can bring many advantages to your body. It is also a great option to be placed on any swelling on the body to be used as a poultice.

Chamomile

Chamomile isn't just an ordinary flower, but it also offers a variety of medicinal advantages. There are endless lists of illnesses which can be treated using the chamomile. The flowers and leaves of chamomile can be prepared in tea to improve the health of the nervous and digestive system. The aroma of chamomile could also help to improve the mood of those struggling with anxiety or stress. It also offers benefits for those who struggle with sleeping. You can add dried chamomile flowers or essential oil into their bath to experience the healing benefits that they require.

Chamomile contains volatile oils , such as chamazulene, farnesene and bisabolol. It also has flavonoids, such as quercimertrin the coumarins, rutin and various types of acids known as plan acid. The volatile oils offer anti-inflammatory and antibacterial properties of the chamomile. This is the reason the leaves and flowers of chamomile can use to heal cuts burns, abrasions, and abrasions as poultice.

Cinnamon

Cinnamon is dried, sloughed bark from the cinnamon tree. It is a wonderful, fragrant spice, which is a source of volatile oils. It also has tannins resin, coumarin, eugenol and mucilage, which make this spice highly effective for treating various ailments.

The cinnamon's tannins have conferred this spice with antimicrobial properties. Infusions of cinnamon essential oil can be a potent natural remedy for athletes foot. Additionally adding cinnamon powder in your favorite drink will not only enhance the flavor of your beverage but also aids in fighting off cold and flu.

Furthermore, using cinnamon in tincture form is an effective method to treat oral yeast infections and other forms of gum conditions like gum disease and oral thrush. In addition it is also an effective treatment in the treatment of Type II diabetes.

The process of grinding cinnamon bark is an excellent method to obtain fresh cinnamon. It is possible to sprinkle the powder in herbal teas or drink the powder in their natural form. Be sure to keep it in a sealed airtight container to preserve its freshness. It is essential to maintain the freshness of cinnamon as the old inventory can diminish its medicinal value.

Eucalyptus

Eucalyptus is a well-known plant utilized to combat colds. In fact, it's among the components used in making the tinctures used to make cough drops and syrups. Part of the plant that is of high therapeutic value is the leaves from which its oils are extracted. The oil has 70 percent pinenes, cineole aromadendrene, sesquiterpene , and cuminaldehyde.

Eucalyptus oil can also be an excellent pain relief for arthritis pain and sore muscles. The calming and menthol effects of eucalyptus are great for improving the health for the respiratory tract particularly those suffering from inflammation of the respiratory tract. The leaves also contain antiseptic qualities.

Eucalyptus leaves are boiled in tea and can be used for steam inhalation to provide aromatherapy. It can also be utilized in aroma lamps or as massage oil. It is also utilized to create herbal baths.

Stinging Nettle

Stinging nettles are an herb that is potent and has been well-known throughout the ages as a potent herbal remedy for incontinence and gout. It's also a versatile plant, as all its parts of the plant can be utilized to treat ailments. The stems, leaves and roots of stinging-nettle include mucilage, ammonia, carbonic acid, and formic acid.

The plant also has anti-inflammatory properties and natural antihistamines, making it excellent for clearing nasal passages, reduce the symptoms of hay fever, and ease allergies. The extracts of its roots are also recognized as effective diuretics. This makes the plant a great remedy for incontinence as well as preventing benign prostate growth in males. Regular consumption of nettle root tea may also safeguard kidneys.

The tea that is made from the leaves of stinging Nettle is an effective herbal treatment for arthritis and gout. As this plant has a high amounts of calcium and Silicon It also helps people suffering from osteoporosis.

Reishi Mushroom

Reishi is well-known as the Chinese name Ling Zhi. The extracts of this fungus are used to treat a variety of ailments in Chinese and Japanese medicine. The components found in the reishi mushrooms can treat many different ailments including anxiety, high blood pressure insomnia, asthma, and bronchitis. Additionally, reishi mushrooms are popular for improving the condition of people suffering from hepatitis as well as other liver ailments. In actual fact, it's well-known to treat liver cirrhosis and fatty fatty liver. It is a drinkable tea or powder form, so that it can easily be mixed into drinks and food.

Coleus

Coleus is a well-known garden plant due to its stunning and vibrant leaves. Its leaves Coleus contain a chemical known as forskolin. This particular compound is believed for its ability to treat those suffering from diabetes, high blood pressure, stomach ulcers and weight gain. The most effective portion of the substance is it's root. It can be used to make tea.

Gastro Tract Issues involving the GI Tract Nausea Bloating, Constipation, Nausea, Diarrhea, Abdominal Pain
Nausea and vomiting

The issue: The need to eliminate waste can arise due to various reasons. It could be due to sensitivity to moving motion (like in cars or boats) as well as a result of something that you consumed or drank, or even the flu. No matter what the reason of the reaction, it's always similar. The first thing you do is sweat, salivate and you both pray and fear you'll vomit so that you can bring an end to your sour feelings. Vomiting and nausea can range from an uneasy stomach feeling to the intense action of vomiting immediately. A person who is distressed by nausea and vomiting symptoms must think about the consumption of an irritable food (i.e. foods that contain toxic substances) or poisoning by an infectious agent like salmonella. Vomiting right after eating is typically followed by excessive salivation that is watery. A few cases of chronic nausea that are low intensity can last for a prolonged period because of persistent low-level food allergies or difficulties with food-related combinations. An anxious person suffering from nausea that is low-level will typically have symptoms that disappear after a diet modification. The vomiting and nausea can also be associated with migraines that are that are caused by food allergies.

The Solution

The most straightforward solution is to surrender

to the desire to cleanse and finish it off. If you're still not at that moment and are looking to "settle your stomach" there are a few ways to go about it, they're:

Warm Cola

To remove the fizz of a drink, you can pour it into two glasses at least a couple of times, and then sip the sugary drink. It's as potent as other drugs such as dimenhydrinate (Dramamine).

Ginger

Add 1 teaspoon of dry ginger powder into one cup of hot water then sip (ginger candy is also a good choice). You can find the powder in the local health food store (HFS). The tea made of ginger is just equally effective as scopolamine pills sold for motion sickness.

Barley

Sip tea made of barley. Cook four tablespoons of barley in a cup of water (1 hour) then strain then add milk, and drink the tea. Consuming the cooked barley can help with the feeling of nausea. Barley is rich in catechins, which can help reduce nausea.

Spices

Try eating a cup of plain yogurt, to which you've added 2 teaspoons of cinnamon and half a teaspoon honey. You can also chew the seeds of cardamom, they'll ease your stomach.

Nose

If you are afraid of eating or drinking anything
isn't enough you're not feeling well, dip a towel in
a warm cup of fennel, chamomile or peppermint.
Spread the moist warm cloth over your stomach.
The aroma and warmth can ease tension in your
abdominal muscles.

Bloating

Bloating may be caused by excess gas in the
digestive tract. It can be due to the inability to the
GI Tract to maintain youthful peristaltic
contractions in the stomach and intestine , or the
insufficient amount of digestive enzymes as well
as bile acids in order to quickly break down food
or both of these. Intestinal gas is formed due to
the fermentation process and also from
swallowing air while eating.

There are many other causes for being bloated. If
you're a woman and your hormones change just
prior to menstrual cycle can result in fluid
retention , and the feeling of being full of gas
(some women gain weight during this time, due
to the retention of water). Another cause is
overindulging in salty pretzels, or tortilla chips.
The salty snacks can hold in the body's fluids.
Other puffiness-promoting agents are:

*Corticosteroid Medicines
*Blood Pressure Lowering Drugs
"Inflammatory Reaction" (everything that includes sunburn, insect bites and.
*Allergies: intolerances to: gluten (in wheat) as well as lactose (in milk)

The Solution

The most common solution to bloating due to the retention of water is a pill, also known as a diuretic. The diuretics encourage the kidneys to eliminate the excess sodium, as well as some water. They also flush out essential minerals like potassium, which fights against the retention of fluids. If you experience occasional bloating, there are other natural methods to flush out excess body fluids. These include:

Mineral-rich Tea

With the help of potassium-rich tea, it is possible to reduce the bloating. Parsley is a great option, as it is high in potassium, and creates pleasant tea. Make a cup of chopped parsley into a glass of hot water (drink only one cup per day).

Asparagus Juice

When you cook or stream asparagus, you can save the water, allow it to cool before drinking it straight. Asparagus drippings make a great diuretic. Other foods that function similarly include watercress, artichoke and watermelon.

Water

Drinking plenty of water can help (8 glasses a day). Food allergies can irritate the digestive tract, causing the body to hold on to fluid. Drinking water can help the kidneys eliminate the irritating substances.

Foods rich in Potassium

Potassium-rich foods fight water retention. The most effective would be:

*Sunflower Seeds

*Dates

*Figs

*Oranges

*Peaches

*Bananas

*Tomatoes

*All leafy green vegetables (even the celery's tops)

Foods that are processed and prepared contain sodium or salt. This helps to retain fluids, and is found in everything from cereal to cheese. Also, look over the food labels with an attentive eye. The goal is to keep your sodium intake to between 1,000 and 2 milligrams (mg). Consider using tangy spices and them to substitute sodium in the diet. Keep in mind that a teaspoon of salt is more than 2,000 mg sodium. Also, try paprika on your popcorn or sprinkle flakes from basil in your beans in place of salt.

Vitamin B6

Bloating can occur if you're deficient in vitamin B6. B6 aids in the metabolism of hormones (including the hormones that trigger premenstrual bleeding). Consider a B-complex supplement instead than taking individual B Vitamin supplements.

Constipation

The issue: Constipation is the decrease in frequency or slowing of the peristalsis (GI Tract contractions), which results in stools that are more difficult to pass. If the GI Tract gets reduced, feces will build up in the colon, causing associated irritation as well as toxic reaction. Spastic colon occurs when the colon expands out of rhythm, causing painful spasms, preventing movements of the stool. There are some who experience constipation that is painful, that are followed by a forceful, bloated and watery stool. Often, it is associated with abdominal cramps.

Constipation is directly connected (in the majority of instances) to eating habits. If you regularly binge on meat, sugar bread, chocolate, bread (although it is okay to have a small amount of dark chocolate is acceptable) as well as alcohol and dairy products is one who suffers regularly with constipation. This diet is not one that is high in fiber. Fiber (plant substances) increases the volume of stool and makes it more soft. This, when it is pressed against the colon's wall triggers peristalsis. The wave-like contractions activate an elimination reaction.

Treatments for pain or high blood pressure excessive stress, eating your food, insufficient fiber in your diet, and a lack of physical exercise all contribute to the infrequent and irregular. The delay in removing the urge (maybe due to the fact that public restrooms are not enjoyable) is not a good idea since the longer stool remains within the colon, the more difficult it becomes (because the water is constantly being absorbed by inside the colon). When you wait for elimination, people's habits change and the cycle continues to feed on itself. In the end, hemorrhoids can cause or worse intestinal issues. In many instances "regularity" is determined by routines and the habits that keep you regularly are good for you. If you regularly make use of laxatives (the common method of treating constipation) your colon will start to depend on them for its task. This is an "bad" habit that can be able to develop.

The colon will turn "lazy" in addition to "weak" and will be unable to function normally without laxative effects. When the colon is transformed to the state of a "lazy colon" and is weak, it requires more and more doses of the laxatives in order to achieve an elimination. This is not a great situation However, there are many natural cures that can help. They include:

The Solution

Water

Everyone agrees that the easiest way to activate the colon is by drinking water...lots of it. For a lazy colon make sure you drink 8 to 10 glasses of water in the span of 24 hours.

Oatmeal

Oatmeal is a wonderful breakfast cereal. Oatmeal is among the food items that have an extremely high amount of water-soluble fiber, also known as mucillage. This is precisely the kind of fiber that is required to eliminate waste regularly. Fruits added in cereal is a benefit. Be careful with butter and sugar as they're not recommended. It is acceptable to cook the oatmeal using water or milk that is nonfat.

Psyllium

Visit your local grocery store or health food shop for psyllium. it's a powdered laxative which contains the ground seeds of psyllium. Psyllium is a mucilaginous. Every day you can add 2 tablespoons of the substance to the large glass of juice or water and drink it prior to when it gets thicker. Drink plenty of fluids throughout the day to prevent obstruction of the intestines (drink at minimum six glasses). Do not take psyllium within 2 hours after taking other medication or supplement. It can hinder their absorption into your bloodstream.

Prunes

Prunes for every ounce are packed with more soluble fiber than all food items we consume. Additionally they contain an organic laxative known as dihydroxyphenyl isatin (raisins also have this natural ingredient however, in a lesser amount). Take a bite of dry prunes and figs or raisins...they are effective.

Dandelion Roots

Fresh dandelion roots contain a natural laxative. This double benefit means that your lawn will look less weedy, and you gain from an effective natural laxative. Remove the entire the dandelion grass from your yard. Use the fresh roots cut up in a salad or infuse the roots in a cup of boiling water for about 10 to 15 minutes. Your neighborhood health store may offer dandelion tea in a packaged form. If you're taking potassium or diuretics consult your physician before taking the dandelion.

Vitamin C

One of the negative side negative effects of excessive vitamin C supplements is diarrhea. If you don't suffer from stomach or kidney problems The side effect can begin as low as 1000 milligrams of buffeted Vitamin C pills every 2 hours. Once you have eliminated the problem, cut back to 500 milligrams per every day.

Magnesium

One of the most popular laxatives is magnesium milk. Deficiency in magnesium can cause constipation. Spinach is high in magnesium. Add it to your diet to get some natural relief.

Potato Juice

Although researchers are unable to pinpoint the reason drinking the juice the vegetables were cooked with is believed to work its magic.

Conserve the potato juice you drank the night before mixing two tablespoons of the juice from potatoes and two tablespoons of honey into the hot water in a cup and drink it before breakfast.

Diarrhea

The Issue: Diarrhea is the increased frequency of bowel movements which can be fluid and loose. If diarrhea becomes more frequent the likelihood of celiac disease is thought to be a possibility. Celiac disorder is a severe disease that permits certain macromolecules to enter the intestinal wall. If blood is present in the stool it is likely that ulcerative colitis has occurred. Insistent bouts of diarrhea may cause nutritional deficiencies because of the poor absorption of vital nutrients. Diarrhoea can be triggered through certain foods that are part of our diet. For some sugar in all forms whether it's fructose, or lactose found in milk, isn't a good choice and may cause digestive distress. Artificial sweeteners, alcohol, anti-acids and megadoses in magnesium and vitamin C may also trigger diarrhea. The same is true for antibiotics that can cause loose stool.

Diarrrhea may also be a sign of more serious health issues like food poisoning, digestive disorders such as IBS. It may also mean that you're not getting the nutrients you need due to diabetes, anemia or thyroid issues or a different related condition.

If your diarrhea is laced by blood, this could indicate an infection or even an actual tumor. It's likely to be a serious issue. There are a variety of non-pharmacological remedies that reduce the amount of waste, and may even solve the issue. Note of caution: If your diarrhea persists for more than 36-48 hours, regardless of your best self-care attempts to stop the illness, it's time to see your doctor (immediately) particularly when your stool appears bloody.

The Solution If you are a lover of travel but are afraid of the repercussions (diarrhea). Make sure you treat yourself with probiotics (good bacteria) prior to your trip. It has been discovered that certain strains of bacteria known as lactobacillus GG (LGG) can prevent travelers from getting diarrhea. The typical dosage is one or two capsules per day in conjunction with food. "Beneficial microbes "...so known as"good bugs" are powerful healing agents that remove those bad bugs that could cause your diarrhea. Consuming dairy products that have lactobacillus acidophilus isn't the most effective method to treat diarrhea. Find lactobacillus acidophilus the form of capsules or liquid at your local health food store, and adhere to the directions on the packaging.
Valerian

Valerian is a plant-based sleep remedy It can help to ease the spasms in your intestines. It's especially effective if you're suffering from constipation in your intestines. Consume one or two capsules of between 100 and 300 milligrams per day for as long as you are experiencing symptoms. As valerian is a sleeping aid, it could cause drowsiness. Therefore, it is recommended to take it prior to going to bed. Do not take valerian if taking another medication, including antidepressants or anti-anxiety drugs...it could affect the absorption.

Slippery Elm Bark

The elm bark of slippery slippery soothes the mucous membranes of bowel, with no or very little adverse negative effects. Add 1/4 teaspoon of the powder made from slippery elm into the applesauce in a cup and eat it three to every day. Add 30 to 40 drops of the tincture into the water in a glass and drink it once every two hours until you stop having diarrhea. Both of these can be purchased at your health food shop.

Burning Diarrhea

Relieve the heat by drinking marshmallow tea. You can find marshmallow tea in your local health food store. Follow the instructions on the packaging to prepare the tea.

Garlic

Garlic is among the most effective ways to combat illnesses, be it diarrhea or flu. When you are sick, take 200-400 milligram capsules 3 times a day. The garlic capsules can be purchased at your local health food store.

Goldenseal

If you suspect that something you consumed is at the source of diarrhea There are three possible causes (all contain bacteria) They include:

*E. Coli

*Giardia

*Salmonella

Goldenseal, a herb that may dry up the mucous membranes of the intestine, could help beat these bugs. This tea can be bitter therefore the best option is capsules. Consume 250 milligrams three times a day until diarrhea eases.

Grapefruit Seed Extract (GSE)

GSE is a substance made up of the seeds and grapefruit's pulp. GSE is able to eliminate any parasite, bacterium, or virus that could be causing your diarrhea. Include two drops in the water in a glass and take it two times a every day. Don't take GSE on its own, as it can eliminate all the colon bacteria which is both bad and good. If you're taking cholesterol-lowering medication be sure to avoid taking GSE.

Abdominal Pain

The Issue: Abdominal pain manifests in various patterns and at different intensities and for a variety of reasons. The reason for this is due to muscles spasms that affect abdominal organs. Extreme cramping pain, which is commonly known as colic, typically results as a result of a strong allergic reaction to food items. The abdominal cramping that occurs around the navel comes due to the small intestine as well as near the sides, the top and the bottom of the lower abdomen. the pain can be traced to the colon. Nearly everyone at some point is likely to experience abdominal discomfort. The majority of causes aren't serious and are easily diagnosed and treated. But, pain may be a sign of serious disease. It is essential to recognize signs that are extreme and be aware of when to contact an emergency physician. The following ailments are able to cause abdominal discomfort:

*Stomach virus

*Menstrual cramps

*Food allergy

*Pelvic inflammation disease

*Hernia

*Kidney stones

*Endometriosis
*Urinary tract infection
*Appendicitis
As can be seen from the list of ailments that could be creating abdominal pain...the person reading the list must be know which ones merit an appointment with a doctor. If you are experiencing abdominal pain associated with any of the following conditions, you should call your physician:
*Fever
Inability to keep food intake down (for many days)
*Can't bowel movements (and your body is vomiting)
*Urinary discomfort or frequent urination.
* The abdomen feels tender pressure
*The abdominal pain can be the consequence of an accident.
The pain is felt for several days.
The Solution - Schedule an appointment for a medical exam
The above indicators indicate an issue with your health which requires treatment as quickly as is possible. But, there are more serious symptoms that need to be taken into consideration, and they include:

*Vomit blood
*Have an unclean stool
*Are having trouble breathing
Are you experiencing pain in your pregnancy?
There are many possible causes for abdomen pain
physician will inquire regarding the source of the
pain. They will ask:
What is the cause of hurt?
The pain is located in the area of the discomfort?
The type of pain...stabbing or the sensation of a
dull ache?
When does the pain begin?
Do you feel that the pain is radiating into other
parts or your body?
What are the medications you are taking?
Are you expecting?
Do any activities alleviate discomfort?
*Have you sustained an injury in the last few
days?
After an initial assessment has been completed
Your doctor is likely to request tests to help
determine the root cause of the discomfort. The
tests you can take include:
*Stool
*Urine
*Blood
*Endoscopy

*X-ray

*Ultrasound

*CT Scan

Treatment of abdominal pain is dependent on the cause. The medical treatment options can range from medicines for inflammation acid Indigestion (Gastro Esophageal Resflux Disease, GERD), or ulcers and antibiotics to treat infections, as well as adjustments in the way you behave to treat abdominal pain that is caused by certain beverages or food items. In certain instances such as appendicitis or hernias, surgery may be required.

In certain cases, abdominal pain may be diagnosed as Irritable Bowel Syndrome (IBS...to be discussed in a subsequent chapter). It isn't clear what triggers the abdominal pain in IBS however it is believed that it is caused by abnormal abdominal muscles...visceral hyper-sensitivity.

Chapter 4: Natural Remedies To Overcome Anxiety

There are many different medications that are prescribed for those suffering from anxiety or panic attacks. They offer a short solution and can help with the issue however when it comes to finding a long-term solution to the issue the medication isn't the ideal option to pursue. Consider, do you really want to continue taking the medication forever? If no, then you may want to consider natural alternatives to help deal with anxiety while offering you a longer-term solution. Natural remedies are superior than prescription drugs in some ways. For instance, they're less potent so there's no risk of harm to any organs in your body. Do you realize that prescribing medication can result in subtle changes in the chemical composition that your body has? Herbal remedies aren't dependent, which means you're not at risk of becoming dependent on them to get better. They do not have major adverse effects or cause you to feel withdrawal symptoms after you quit using the products. That's a huge advantage when you look at modern anxiety medication like benzodiazepines, which can cause dependence. Another benefit of using herbal remedies is that they do not alter your mood, unlike other anxiety drugs. You'll not feel tired and fatigued for the remainder of the day following taking the medication. Since they're not as powerful the reaction time is similar and you will not be sluggish. What's more what's the best way to take advantage of the treatment if you only want to do is lay in bed after having it?

Are you interested in giving herbal remedies a shot to aid in reducing anxiety? Here's a brief list of most popular herbs used to treat anxiety. Be sure to check with your physician prior to using any of them in order to make sure you're not allergic to.

Kava Kava Root

Roots of Kava are the source of its roots. Kava plant are commonly utilized to create a type of tea that has anesthetic and sedative qualities. It is used extensively in areas like Polynesia, Vanuatu, Hawaii and even a few parts of Micronesia. It has also been proven by studies that it could be an effective alternative for treating anxiety that is chronic and chronic and panic attacks. It has a lower chance of dependency , and even lesser chance of having any side negative effects. There is a prescribed dosage, so consult your doctor or natural medicine practitioner for guidance on how to make use of it.

Valerian Root

It is recognized for its relaxing effects and is employed to promote more restful sleep. It is usually prescribed to sufferers of insomnia, as it assists them to get to sleep more easily, without the risk of dependence. The same effect of calming can be utilized to reduce anxiety and stress. It is able to relax the body and mind effortlessly. Many people mix it with meditation, or any other exercise, like yoga. It is not known to cause any major adverse effects, but not take it with alcohol.

Passion Flower

The effects of this supplement are similar to Kava however, they are less noticeable. It has been proven by research that it aids in alleviating moderate anxiety. This means you can have a more gentle option when managing the issue rather than choosing the more powerful alternative. It is perfect for a simple relaxation as well. If you're looking for a way to unwind after a long day, but tension doesn't be able to go away from your thoughts and body, take one of these and you'll be more calm and relaxed without the sleepiness.

St. John's Wort

This specific herb has been used to treat mental health issues for centuries now. If you suffer of depression, this may offer relief- it is the same for people who are suffering from anxiety attacks or chronic clinical anxiety. It can help relax the mind and easing any tension within the body. For those who suffer from insomnia, it could assist in getting a better night's sleep. Because it's an all-natural treatment it is not a risk of dependence.

Chapter 5: Common Herbal Medicines

Acai
Helps with weight loss , and to reduce the
accumulation in dental plaque.

Agrimony
It is used to soothe sore throats. It is also utilized
to loosen the bowels. It can also be utilized to
reduce fevers as well as a range of digestive
problems.

Alfalfa
Also known as "the food that started it all" Alfalfa
is full of minerals and vitamins, and an abundance
of protein. It can be used to treat arthritis, lower
cholesterol levels and help with digestion issues.
It also assists in helping to build your immune
system.

Aloe vera
The leaves are used to heal burns, cuts and
various skin conditions.

Amla
High in Vitamin C, it is used to treat urinary tract
infections, reduce joints inflammation, treat
fevers and regulate blood sugar levels.

Angelica
Helps to alleviate digestive problems such as
flatulence, loss of appetite, and menopausal-

related issues in women, it can also be used to assist those suffering from arthritis and respiratory issues.

Anise

Typically, when it is made into tea, it tastes similar to licorice. It is utilized to enhance digestion in the body, relieve flatulence, treat common cough, and help reduce bad breath.

Arnica

It is a form of ointment that it is used to treat bruises, sprains and muscles that are sore. It is also known for its anti-septic and anti-inflammatory properties.

Ashwagandha

The herb is utilized to reduce stress and boost your immune system. Its seeds plant are well-known for their anti-inflammatory properties and sedative effects as well.

Astragalus

It is considered to be one among the most sought-after herbs in Chinese treatment it has been employed for over 2 millennia to lower blood pressure, and to treat respiratory infections of the upper respiratory tract. It has been proven to boost general energy levels, decrease excessive sweating, diarrhea, or even the formation of ulcers.

Bacopa

For thousands of years, it has been used as a powerful stimulant for the brain the herb has been shown to be a permanent boost to the human brain's memory. It is being investigated at present as a possible component of the treatment of Alzheimer's disease, Parkinson's and ADHD.

Bearberry

Most often, it is consumed as tea It is utilized for treating urinary tract infection as well as the inflammation it creates.

Bee Balm

Typically, it is consumed as a kind or tea. This plant is known to help ease digestion issues, flatulence and colic. It's made to cause sweating to reduce fevers.

Bee Pollen

It is rich in Vitamins, enzymes as well as amino acids it's easily digested , allowing the body to absorb the top quality nutrients we need to flourish.

Bilberry

For thousands of years, it was used by healers throughout Europe Bilberry has been used to treat diarrhea, diabetes or stomach cramps. The fruit has also been utilized to treat night blindness.

Black Cherry

It has been used over the years as a way to treat a recurring cough. It is usually created into a tea from syrup. It is also utilized to treat an unsatisfactory appetite, throat sores, and pneumonia.

Black Cohosh

It has been utilized as an excellent remedy for fatigue and tuberculosis. It was first employed to treat fatigue by Cherokee Indians. It can also help with sore throatsand rheumatism and menstrual issues for women.

Boneset

It was initially used to treat Native Americans to treat the common flu and cold This herb has numerous beneficial properties. It is utilized to treat constipation, loss of appetite and malaria. It also helps with typhoid, malaria dengue, cholera and arthritis.

Borage

In the treatment of infections, it also assists by reducing fevers as well as aiding in the inflammation of mucous membranes in the case of a bad cold.

Boswellia

It has been utilized by healers of the past for over 2 millennia to treat ailments like diabetes and rheumatism, as well as cardiovascular diseases as well as asthma, and fevers. It can also help relieve joint pain.

Buchu

The herb is believed to stimulate tonics and also acts as a diuretic. It is commonly used to treat the urinary tract infection. It can also be used to help the treatment of kidney stones and gout and arthritis.

Burdock

The herb was first utilized in the early Greeks to treat wounds and infections. wounds. It is rich in minerals and vitamins it was used to treat psoriasis Eczema, live ulcers, and also to increase stamina and energy levels.

Butterbur

It is used to treat the treatment of fevers, eliminate intractable intestinal parasites. It can also treat urinary tract issues and coughs that are common.

Calendula

Helps with swelling, jaundice as well as problems with liver and stomach, and can even trigger menstrual flow for women.

Cascara Sagrada

The first time it was used, it was in the past by Native Americans as a common laxative for constipation. It also helps with other digestive problems, hemorrhoids, colitis and jaundice.

Catnip

It is used to treat irritations on scalps, restlessness bruises, gas and common cough. It as well as to treat colic, common cold and flu and diarrhea.

Cats claw

It has been used for many years to make an ingredient used in cooking recipes used to can treat and prevent illness.

Cayenne

The use of this herb is to relieve pain and to treat infections. Also , it helps reduce arthritis pain and toothache.

Chamomile

The use of this herb was for centuries by Egyptians to ease the symptoms of fever and chills The herb is widely used in our modern times. It is helpful in relieving anxiety, heartburn, bloating and stomach indigestion.

Chaparral

Helps with common cold and flu as well as to ease digestive problems and intestinal issues. It is an antioxidant that is powerful which is being researched to treat cancer.

Chaste Tree

Since the beginning of time it has been utilized to assist with menstrual issues and encourage normal menstrual cycle. Nowadays, it is frequently used to ease PMS symptoms.

Chicory

It is used to aid digestion, and treat nausea, inflammation, and common cold.

Cinnamon rose

Utilized in the making from rose hip syrup which is high in Vitamin C.

Clove

It is used to treat stomach upsets Also, clove oils can be utilized to treat common toothache.

Clubmoss

It has been used by healers from the beginning of time for over two thousand years. It was used as a purgative as well as a laxative. It was utilized to treat fevers and to reduce bleeding from wounds. Nowadays, it is used to treat stomach issues and urinary problems, kidney issues, and even skin problems.

Comfrey

This herb has been utilized since the days that of ancient Greeks to reduce bleeding. It and was also consumed as a tea to alleviate the symptoms of diarrhea and bronchitis.

Cordyceps

This is a powerful tonic that improves power and endurance. It can also treat bronchitis asthma, and common cold.

Dandelion

The herb has been used for many thousands of years to be used to treat digestive problems. It was often used to combat breast inflammation to stimulate milk flow.

Dong Quai

In the name of female Ginseng in China The herb is popular among women because it's known to be a cure for menstrual issues and reduces pain in menstrual cycles and bleeding.

Echinacea

An herb that is widely used to treat colds and flus It is an excellent herb to help build the immune system.

Eucalyptus

Helps to ease symptoms of colds and cough.

Fo-Ti

The longevity herb has been used in China for quite a while and is very popular among old gentlemen. It is believed to turn hair that is gray back to its original shade. It also aids in the strength of hips as well as the back.

Ginger

It is used to ease nausea.

Ginko Biloba

This herb boosts the circulation of blood to the brain, and also increases the quantity of oxygen that is delivered to brain cells. It improves cognitive capacity and memory.

Ginseng

In its capacity as an adaptogen it's utilized to aid the body to protect itself from stress. The most popular use for it is to boost the immune system stronger and improve overall physical endurance.

Gotu Kola

The herb was originally used to ease congestions and other respiratory problems It is also well-known for its healing properties that assist in healing wounds in a rapid manner. It is widely used to treat memory loss as well as for varicose veins too.

Gynostemma

This herb has the ability to put the body in an improved state of equilibrium. It shields the mind and body from the negative effects of stress . It also helps individuals build up their physical power.

Holy Basil

Reduces anxiety, depression, and stress. This herb

can be very effective in promoting overall well-being.

Kava

It was first used by the inhabitants of the Pacific islands It has been used over the years to treat anxiety. It is known for its calming properties that can make anyone, even stressed people in a more positive mood.

Korean Ginseng

This herb can help people manage stress more effectively. Its energy-boosting properties aid in creating more focus, improve endurance and strength, and keep from fatigue.

Lemon balm

It is used as a sleep and digestion aid.

Lemongrass

The herb is used to treat a wide range of problems, including cancer, digestive issues and gas, pain, fevers and anxiety, flu and sleep issues.

Licorice

It is used to treat stomach ulcers and bronchitis, and those with common sore throats. as well as to combat infections caused by viruses such as hepatitis, for instance.

Mane of Lion Mane

Utilized to strengthen immunity, the herb assists in improving digestion and colon health, and also aids in easing anxiety and depression.

Lycium Fruit

In the last hundred of centuries by Chinese the Chinese, this herb is known for its delicious health benefits. The fruit of the Lycium plant are among the healthiest foods on the planet Earth. They are loaded with minerals and vitamins. It can improve overall health.

Maca

This herb can help the body to deal with stress. Its roots are very abundant in vitamins, minerals amino acids, and healthy fats. It is widely regarded in the modern world as an superfood. It can help increase the stamina of a person, boost energy levels, and soothe the nervous system.

Milk Thistle

This herb is excellent in protecting the gallbladder as well as the liver. It does this by detoxifying the blood. It's also been shown to aid in treatment for cancer.

Maitake

This mushroom is rich in antioxidants minerals and vitamins which have been found to treat auto immune disorders and cancer.

Rhodiola

It is popular in Russia the world of astronauts and athletes have utilized this herb to boost endurance and power. It helps the body use less oxygen. It also helps improve the mind and retention of memories.

Saw Palmetto

The herb is commonly utilized by males older than 40. It can help treat urinary pain. It also assists in the treatment of male pattern baldness.

Schizandra

Consuming this herb can help people to cope with mental and physical tensions more easily. It's packed with nutrients that will provide those who drink it energy. It has also been proved to provide great benefits for skin in addition.

Shilajit

With a wealth of vitamins and minerals The herb is well-known for its ability to improve longevity overall.

Siberian Ginseng

The herb is regarded as an effective stress reliever and boost in energy. It has been used for many years as an adaptogen that helps help balance the body.

Skullcap

The herb has been used for hundreds of years to assist in sleeping. It eases anxiety and anxiousness. It helps in reducing cholesterol, blood pressure and muscles spasms.

St. John's Wort

The anti-depressant properties of the drug are well-known It allows serotonin to remain in the place it's needed to relieve anxiety and feelings of depression.

Suma

This herb boosts stamina as well as strength. It also aids in reducing stress. It is also known to improve the immune system of humans and boost the immune system.

Tea oil from trees

As an antibacterial or antifungal agent.

Turmeric

Traditional Chinese medicine that assists in menstrual cycle regulation as well as relieving arthritis pain. improving liver function and digestion.

Thyme

It is used to treat common cough and bronchitis.

Valerian Root

This herb has been used for many decades to help treat sleeplessness and decrease stress. It has also been proven to be extremely effective in combating anxiety-related symptoms.

Yarrow

The herb is utilized as astringent, stimulant, and tonic. It is renowned for its aromatic properties.

Chapter 6: Natural Remedies For Mild Infections

Common Cold

The cold may be one of the most simple and least dangerous illnesses that you may experience at times however, it can be an illness that is crippling. Unfortunately the cure for cold hasn't been found and the best we can do is ease the symptoms that cause the cold to be uncomfortable as well as causing congestion. aid the immune system in fighting to fight back.

* Mullein. Mullein tea is a natural remedy which alleviate nasal congestion by causing your body to eliminate the mucus build-up. For you to enjoy it as a tea it is necessary to infuse 1 tablespoon of dried mullein leaf and one teaspoon of its dried flower in a glass filled with boiling water for about 15 minutes. Be sure to strain the tea properly, as it has tiny hairs that could irritate your throat and mouth. Limit your use to three times every day.

* Chicken noodles soup. This chicken soup legend is trueand it can assist you in getting over colds fast. The secret behind the soup lies in the ingredients that are proven to boost your

immune system. It can also flush out congestion and ease irritations. These include carrots, celery, onions as well as hot broth. It is possible to make soup any way you'd like, but do not use the soups available in the stores.

* Garlic. Garlic is antibacterial as well as anti-inflammatory properties which help to cleanse your airways of congestion. Incorporate a large amount of garlic into your meals or make an herbal tea with garlic by boiling five garlic cloves in one cup of water, and then letting it infuse for up to 6 minutes.

Coughs

Cough typically occurs in conjunction with or following a bout of cold, which makes it even difficult to bear. It's also embarrassing when you're forced to cough up and cry when you are in public areas. To get rid of cough, follow these steps:

Honey is a good option. Research has proven that honey is an efficient demulcent that forms soft protection to the lining of the throat, which reduces irritation. Simply take 3 tablespoons pure organic honey every day.

Drink a cup of ginger tea. Ginger is an effective natural stimulant that is effective in removing sweat from the body. Take it while it's warm and steaming hot.

* Drink tea with thyme. Thyme is a source of components that can help in relaxing and soothing the airways and lungs. Four sprigs fresh thyme and crush them gently. Allow them to sit in a glass filled with boiling drinking water for about 15 mins, then take three times per day.

Inhale steam inhaling essential oils. Steam aids in breaking down mucous and phlegm that is stubborn to break down and essential oils such as those of eucalyptus or peppermint aid in clearing the airways and eliminating the infection. Simply take an ice bath with 2 drops of oil from peppermint, and two drops of eucalyptus oil. Put your face on the bowl and breathe in the steam, but be sure that it's not hot enough to cause your face to be scalding. This is helpful for colds too.

Sore Throat

A sore throat can be difficult, and can be a problem when the majority of your time, you need to speak. Colds, coughs and sore throat all are all part of the same category of diseases and that is the reason why treatment for the two other ailments are effective in treating sore throats. Other natural remedies to relieve sore throat are:

* Apple cider vinegar. AVC is acidic and can kill the bacteria inside your throat. Simply mix one teaspoon of it into one cup of warm water and drink it, or gargle prior to drinking it.

* Gargle with warm salt. Gargling salty water helps reduce the swelling of the throat's membranes and relieve pain because salt draws out the water. Mix one teaspoon of salt into one cup of warm water and gargle it three times a every day.

* Pomegranate juice. It has an astringent effect that reduces swelling and therefore reduce the pain. Two glasses of organic pomegranate juice that is unsweetened juice daily be sure you rinse it out prior to drinking it.

First Aid Ointment

When you experience an accident, you must immediately seek out creams and lotions that are chemical and comprised of chemicals. Even without them, you can still provide first aid using your pantry and the natural elements as your kit of healing.

Plantain Ointment

Plantain is an unwelcome weed for some, however, it is a potent herb which are ideal for the first-aid treatment of wounds, bites, stings as well as allergies, rashes sunburns and various skin conditions. For making plantain ointment all you need is these ingredients:

* 4 oz. olive oil infused with dried plantain leaves
* 1 oz. Beeswax
* 5 drops Vitamin E (oil)
Three drops oil containing peppermint
* 2 Mason jars

How to Prepare

1. To infuse olive oil make sure to fill the dried Mason jar (a quarter of a quart) by adding dried leaves of plantain and olive oil. Secure the seal. Place the jar inside the crock-pot, with a layer of towels on the bottom. Fill it with water until it covers the top of the container. Then, set it to remain warm for two days.

2. To make the ointment add beeswax, oil and strained in a pan set over a the flame at a low temperature. Stir until it has melted. Incorporate to the Vitamin E oil and the peppermint oil. Stir. Transfer the mixture to a dry Mason jar , and allow to stand for a day or two to firm. Reuse as

required.

Chapter 7: Herbs To Treat Common Ailments

Allspice

Indigestion, Flatulence, Joint & Muscle Pain, Bruising, Laxative, Vomiting, Gum Problems, Fever, Heavy Menstruation

Anti-inflammatory, Anti-fungal, Anti-bacterial

Cautions:

* If you are pregnant or nursing Allspice can be used in small amounts

* Avoid taking for 2 weeksprior to and after the surgery because it may slow the process of clotting blood which could cause problems with the surgery as well as post surgery healing

If you are sensitive skin, you must conduct a skin test since it could trigger an allergic reaction.

* Do not take if are taking an anticoagulant medication

Basil

Respiratory Problems, Allergies Coughs Anxiety, Stress Coughs Asthma, Flu, Bronchitis, Earache, Headache Stomach Upsets Fever Insomnia,

Ringworm
Anti-inflammatory, Anti-spasmodic, Anti-bacterial

Precautions:* Avoid when you are pregnant or nursing.
* Do not take any medication for two weeks prior to and after the surgery because it could slow blood clotting which could cause problems with the surgery as well as post surgery healing
* Don't take if you are taking an anticoagulant medication

Bay
Flatulence, Stimulates Sweating Dandruff Joint Pain Muscular Pain Cramps Boils
Anti-spasmodic, Anti-bacterial
Cautions:
Avoid if you are you are breastfeeding or pregnant.
* Do not take it for two weeks prior to and after

surgery, as it could reduce the central nervous system that could cause complications if mixed with anaesthetic.

Do not use if you suffer from diabetes since Bay may affect the levels of blood sugar

* Do not take sedatives if you are taking them.

* Do not take pain medications

Calendula

Minor Wounds and Cuts Burns, Bruises, Stings Minor Skin Rashes Itching, minor skin infections Menstrual Cramps, sore Throat and Conjunctivitis. Haemorrhoids Varicose Veins and Inflammation Mild Sedative Antiseptic and anti-inflammatory

Cautions:

* Do not consume if you are breastfeeding or pregnant.

* Do not take antidepressants or sedatives

* Do not take it for two weeks before and after surgery , as it may cause extreme Drowsiness when combined with surgery drugs

* Allergy Warning Avoid Calendula If you're allergic to marigolds, daisies, chrysanthemums , or any other plants belonging to the family of ragweed

Cayenne Pepper (NOT SEEDS)
Ulcers, Circulation, Boost Organ Strength,
Shingles, Nausea, Immune System, Digestive
Disorders, Herpes, Pleurisy, Psoriasis,
Rheumatism, Arthritis
Anti-inflammatory, Natural Fat Burner
Cautions:
Avoid if you are you are breastfeeding or
pregnant.
* Allergy Tips Avoid if you're intolerant to
banana's kiwi's or bananas avocado, chestnuts
and avocado latex
* Do not use Cayenne Pepper cures for longer
than 1 to 2 weeks at any one period of time.
* Do not take if you are taking anticoagulants,
antacids or anti-coagulants.
Do not use if you are taking any medications
containing Theophylline, (prescribed for
respiratory conditions like asthma)
Do not apply directly to the face of a newborn
child.
* Do not apply on skin that is broken.

Chamomile

Indigestion Nausea, Menstrual Pain, Sinusitis, Eczema, Vomiting, Sore Throat, Nappy Rash, Liver/Gallbladder, Sore Nips, Gum Problems, Cuts, Haemorrhoids

Cautions:

* Do not drink when you are pregnant or nursing.

* Allergy Tips Avoid Calendula If you're sensitive to marigolds, daisies, chrysanthemums and any other plant belonging to the family of ragweeds.

Chickweed

Constipation, Stomach Upset Bowel Problems, Psoriasis, Obesity, Asthma, Muscle and Joint Boils, Pain Abscesses, Ulcers

Cautions:

* Little is known about the use of chickweed during the mother and baby, so it is advised to avoid the use of chickweed during these periods.

Chilli Pepper

Digestive Upset, Hangover Increase Circulatory System Colds, Rheumatism Arthritis Muscular and

Joint Pain, Cluster Headache, Rhinitis, Heartburn, Bowel Problems, Hay Fever, Cramps, Laryngitis, Fever, Nausea, Migraine, Colic
Anti-inflammatory, Anti-spasmodic
Cautions:
* Could cause irritation to skin that is sensitive If you are concerned, do an initial patch test
* Do not apply it to the skin of infants and children
* Do not consume if nursing or pregnant.
* Do not consume for 2 weeksprior to and after the surgery since it may result in an increased amount of bleeding.
* Do not take this if you are you are taking anticoagulant medicine or medications to treat high blood pressure.
* Do not use if you are taking any Theophylline medication
* If you're an addict it is not recommended to utilize Chilli Pepper treatments as they react with cocaine and could cause heart attacks.

Cinnamon
Stomach Cramp Nausea, Stomach Cramp
Digestive Issues, Intestinal Problems Indigestion

Balances Blood Sugar, Increased appetite, bloating Incontinence, Colds Impotence, Menstrual Issues and High Blood Pressure Anti-microbial, Anti-inflammatory, Anti-spasmodic

Cautions:

* Do not drink breastfeeding or if you are pregnant.

* Do not use if diabetic. Cinnamon can make blood sugar drop

* Use with caution if are suffering from liver disease.

Avoid for two months prior to or after surgery

Cloves

Localised Anaesthetic and Digestive Aid Nausea Toothache, Catarrh, Mild Virus Premature Ejaculation Anal Fissures Toothache and Flatulence. Coughs Gingivitis Expectorant, Anti-Viral, Anti-inflammatory

Cautions:

• Do not take if you are pregnant or nursing

* Not recommended on children under the age of

* Reduces blood clotting, so don't use if you have a condition that restricts blood clotting.

Avoid for 2 days prior and after surgery
* Do not take if you are taking anticoagulant
medications.

Coriander
Pain Relief and Digestive Disorders IBS,
Constipation IBS and stimulates the appetite
Muscle Spasms, Fungal Diseases Haemorrhoids
and Toothache. Worms, Joint Pain Nausea
Anti-inflammatory, Anti-spasmodic
Cautions:
* Always conduct the test on your skin if have
sensitive skin. Coriander can trigger symptoms
similar to an allergic reaction.
* Increases the sensitivity to the sun
* Do not consume when you are pregnant or
nursing.
Avoid if you're sensitive to caraway, aniseed,
fennel, or dill
Avoid if you're diabetic. Coriander may cause a
decrease of blood sugar levels.
* Avoid for two days prior and immediately
following surgery

Cumin

Indigestion Morning Sickness Nausea Diarrhoea, Muscle Cramps, Insomnia, Colic, Flatulence and increases Libido
Muscle Relaxant
Cautions:
* Do not consume if you are pregnant or nursing.
* Avoid for two days prior and after surgery
* Do not take if you are diabetic as Cumin may cause a decrease of blood sugar levels.
* Do not take anticoagulants if you are taking them.

Dandelion
Toxillitis Urinary infection, increased appetite, flatulence, Stomach upset and constipation
Arthritis
Cautions:
* Do not consume when you are pregnant or nursing.
Avoid if you are allergic the ragweed plant or any other plants belonging to the family of ragweed
* Do not take any medicine that is altered by the liver , such as acetaminophen and atorvastatin (Lipitor) diazepam (Valium) digoxin, the entacapone (Comtan) and estrogen, Irinotecan (Camptosar) as well as lamotrigine (Lamictal) and

Lorazepam (Ativan) and lovestatin (Mevacor)
meprobamate morphine and Oxazepam (Serax),
* Do not take if you are you are taking diuretics.
* Do not take if you are taking antibiotics.

Dill
Diagestion Colic insomnia and colds and Flu, high
Cholesterol and loss of appetite mild infection,
urinary problems Muscle Spasms, Flatulence
Fever, Sleep Disorders Coughs, Bronchitis,
Anti-spasmodic
Cautions:
* Dill could cause irritation to skin sensitive to so
make sure you do an initial patch test prior to
making use of
* Do not consume if pregnant or nursing
Avoid if you are you are sensitive to coriander,
caraway and fennel. any other family of carrots.
* Dill could decrease blood sugar levels, therefore
avoid it if you're diabetic.
Avoid for two months prior to or after surgery
Avoid taking any medicine that has lithium

Echinacea
The common cold, Vaginal Yeast Infections, Ear

Infections and Anxiety Herpes, Gingivitis, HPV, Flu, Tonsillitis, Warts Urinary Infection and Migraine and Chronic Fatigue Syndrome, Fibromyalgia, Hay Fever, Eczema, Stings, ADHD Anti-viral

Cautions:

* Do not consume if pregnant or breastfeeding

Please do not apply to children who are less than 12 years old

Conduct an examination patch to test for Echinacea can trigger allergy manifestations when applied directly to skin

* Do not use those who suffer from the Auto Immune disorder

Do not take this medication if you are using a medication that is modified by your liver or the body.

Do not use if you are taking medication to weaken the immune system.

Feverfew

Irritable Bowel Syndrome, Arthritis Itching Arthritis Psoriasis, Fever, Allergies Irregular menstrual Cycle, Asthma, Vomiting dizziness, cold

Cautions:

Avoid if you are pregnant or breastfeeding.

* Stay away from if you are have an allergy to ragweed or other plants in the family of ragweeds.
* Avoid for two days prior and after surgery
Avoid using any medication that is anticoagulant. Beware if you are taking medicines that are affected by the liver

Fennel
Colic, Colitis, Constipation, Menstrual Cramps, Upset Stomach, Digestive Issues, Mild Stomach Cramps, Bloating, Flatulence, Bronchitis
Anti-spasmodic
Cautions:
* Fennel can cause skin irritation Always perform an examination of the patch
Avoid breastfeeding during pregnancy and while nursing
* Make use of for 1 week at a stretch in the treatment of children.
* Do not take the product if you suffer from an imbalance of oestrogen or you are taking any medication that contains Oestrogen.
Do not use if you are you are taking anticoagulant medications or have any other issues that interfere in blood clotting.

* Do not take if you are you are allergic to carrots or any other plant in the family of carrots.
* Do not take if you are you are taking contraceptive medications.
Do not take when using antibiotics.

Garlic
Reduces blood pressure, Reduces Cholesterol and ringworm. Genital Fungal Infections, Athletic Foot, Pain triggered from poor circulation, colds, sore Muscles The Corns, Inflammation of the stomach
Anti-fungal Immune Boosting, Anti-bacterial anti-microbial, anti-viral
Cautions:
* Use only in small amounts if nursing or pregnant.
* Can cause irritation and irritation if applied to young or sensitive skin
* Use for a week at a time in the case of children under age 1.
* Lowers Blood Pressure, be sure to avoid it the following if you are suffering from low blood pressure
If you are taking an anticoagulant medication, as garlic can result in an increased risk of bleeding

Do not use if you are taking an antacid medicine or have an intestinal disorder

* Avoid taking medicinal doses garlic for two months prior and immediately following surgery
* Avoid taking medication recommended to treat HIV or AIDS

Avoid taking contraceptive pills.

* Do not use if you are taking medications that are affected by liver function

Ginger

Headaches, Arthritis and Arthritis, as well as Nausea, and Digestive Upset. Dizziness, Morning Sickness Menstrual Motion Sickness, Pain and High Cholesterol Muscular Pain Migraine, Rheumatoid arthritis, Colds and Flu, loss of appetite

Immune Boosting, Anti-bacterial, Anti-viral

Cautions:

* If you are pregnant or breastfeeding the ginger can be considered safe in small amounts, but always consult with your physician or midwife prior to making use of a ginger-based treatment for medicinal purposes.
* Ginger can reduce blood sugar levels, so beware if you are diabetic.

* Ginger could result in a decrease in blood clotting, so stay away from it when you're taking any anticoagulant medication
Do not take taking this medication if you suffer from a blood pressure issue

Lemon Balm
Colds, Calming the digestive System, Cramp & Muscle Spasms Headaches, Lower Fever Anxiety, insomnia, Colic, Dementia, Stomach Upsets, Stress Restlessness, Depression, IBS, Menstrual Cramps The toothache, the nervous Stomach, ADHD
Anti-fungal, Anti-bacterial, Anti-spasmodic
Cautions:
* Avoid when taking anti-depressants or sedative drugs
Avoid if you are you are pregnant or breastfeeding.
* Use only in small amounts and for short time periods in the treatment of children

Marjoram
Sinusitis Congestion, Hay Fever, Asthma, Indigestion, Lightheadedness, Headache, Coughs,

Stomach Pain Sleepiness, Colds, Nervous Disorders, Colic, Liver Problems, Menopause, Menstrual Problems and Nerve Pain. Muscular Discomfort and Sprains. Sleep Disorders
Cautions:
* Do not consume if you are breastfeeding or pregnant.
* Avoid using on children younger than 12 years old.
* Reduces the rate of blood clotting. don't use if you're using an anti-coagulant medication.
* Avoid if sensitive to mint, lavender oregano, basil the hyssop plant and sage
* Do not take medication if you are diabetic.
* Marjoram could cause stomach ulcers to become more severe.
Avoid those who suffer from urinary tract issues as Marjoram can trigger an excess release of fluids from these areas.
Do not take medication the following if you are suffering from any kind of seizures.
Don't use it for two weeks prior to or following surgery.

Nutmeg
Anxiety and Depression, Muscle Relaxant and

Digestive Disorders and improves Memory,
Kidney Disease, Diarrhoea and Muscular Joint
pain
Anti-inflammatory, Anti-septic, Anti-bacterial
Cautions:
If taken in excessive quantities, nutmeg could
trigger psychoactive and hallucinatory reactions.
In small amounts
* Do not consume if breastfeeding or if you are
pregnant.

Oregano
Localised Anaesthetic Anxiety and Nervous
disorders, Toothache, Gum Problems and
Digestion. high Cholesterol, Asthma, Bronchitis,
Coughs, Indigestion, Bloating, Arthritis,
Headaches, Menstrual Cramps
Analgesic, Anti-inflammatory
Cautions:
Do not use this method if you are breastfeeding
or are pregnant.
Avoid for 2 months prior to or after surgery
* Do not take any precautions those who suffer
from diabetes
Avoid if you're allergic to plants belonging to the
Lamiaceae family, which includes lavender,

hyssop and basil mint, marjoram, and sage.
* Do not use if are taking any medication that has Lithium

Paprika
Digestive issues, increases energy levels, Rheumatoid Arthritis, Fibromyalgia and The Back Pain, Rhinitis, Cluster Headaches, Heartburn, Hay Fever, IBS, Toothache, Fever, Colic, Nausea, high Cholesterol migraine, muscle spasms, and Cramps Laryngitis
Anti-inflammatory, Anti-oxidant, Anti-bacterial, Anti-spasmodic
Cautions:
* Do not use on children under 12 years old
* Do not consume breastfeeding or if you are pregnant.
* Do not apply to damaged skin
* Avoid for two days prior and after surgery
* Do not take if you are you are taking Theophylline or anti-coagulant medication.
* Avoid if you're taking medications for high blood pressure.

Peppermint

Insomnia and Insomnia, Upset Stomach
Indigestion Insomnia, Upset Stomach, Indigestion
Tension, Colds, Cramp, Diarrhoea, Nausea,
Coughs, Relaxes Muscles, IBS, Heartburn,
Migraine, Tension Headache, Itching, Stress
Anti-spasmodic, Anti-bacterial, Anti-virus
Cautions:

* Avoid using if you're taking medicines that
contain Cyclosporine
* Use only in small quantities in case you are
pregnant or breastfeeding and for a limited time
period
* Do not take this medication if you are you suffer
from diarrhoea.
* Don't use if you're using a medication that has
been affected by liver function
* Do not take antacids if you are taking
medication
* Do not use on children who are under 10 years
of age.

Peppermint may cause adverse effects, including
heartburn and allergic reactions like headache,
flushing and mouth sores.

Rosemary

Localised Anaesthetic and Digestive Issues
Headaches, Colds and Depression, which
promotes hair Growth Indigestion, Stress, Gout
Coughs and Arthritis. Eczema
Analgesic, Anti-spasmodic, Anti-bacterial
Cautions:
* Do not take if you are allergic to aspirin.
Don't use it if you are you're pregnant or nursing
Avoid if you have blood clotting or seizures

Saffron

(DO NOT MISTAKE for MEADOW SAFFRON, which
is poisonous.)
Depression PMS, Asthma, Erectile Dysfunction,
Psoriasis Coughs, Insomnia, Flatulence and
premature Ejaculation and Muscle pain
Cautions:
* Do not use for longer than six weeks.
* Excessively high doses and long-term use may
result in poisoning, accompanied by symptoms
such as eye and skin jaundice, dizziness; vomiting
and bloody diarrhoea. The lips bleeding, nose and
numbness.
* Avoid if you are pregnant or breastfeeding

* Saffron may affect your mood so be careful if have mood or personality disorders.
Avoid if you are you are allergic to any plant from families like Olea, Lolium or Salsola family
* Saffron may affect the heart rate, so stay clear the spice if you suffer from heart conditions
* Do not take this medication when you have blood pressure issues

Sage
Stress-related illness, depression, Sore Throat, Coughs and Alzheimer's as well as any other memory-related disorder, Cold Sores and High Cholesterol and Menopausal symptoms, Sunburn, Stomach Pain, Asthma, Flatulence, Insomnia, Excessive Sweating
Diuretic, Anti-septic, Anti-spasmodic, Anti-fungal, Anti-inflammatory
Cautions:
Avoid if you are nursing or pregnant.
* Do not use if are diabetic.
* Do not use any medication if you have an hormonal disorder
* Do not use if have a problem with blood pressure
Do not take medication if you suffer from seizures

or are taking any medication that is anti-
convulsant.
* Do not take if you are taking sedative medicine

Tarragon (Mugwort)
Localised Anaesthetic, Digestive aid It stimulates
circulation, Toothache Appetizer Stimulant
Vomiting, Nausea, Menstrual Problems and
Retention of Water
Analgesic
Cautions:
* Do not drink when you are pregnant or nursing.
* Can slow blood clotting. Do not take if you are
taking any anticoagulant medication.
Avoid if you are you are sensitive to any plant
belonging to the family of ragweed
Please avoid using for two weeks prior to or
following surgery.

Thyme
Stomach Upset Coughs and Muscles Relaxes
Wounds that are open and cut, Catarrh,
Bronchitis, Alopecia, Colic, Inflammation of the

mouth, Tongue and Tonsils

Expectorant, Anti-microbial, Anti-septic

Cautions:

* Use in very small quantities for children under the age of 12 or nursing or pregnant.

Avoid if you are sensitive to any plant belonging to the Lamiaceae family, such as oregano

* Can slow the clotting process Beware if you're taking any anticoagulant medication.

* Avoid for two days prior and after surgery

* Avoid if you are suffering from any hormonal disorder

Turmeric

Digestive Upset Boost Immune Systems, Pain Relief, Crohn's Disease, Alzheimer's, Gingivitis Stomach Ulcers IBS, Cancer, Rheumatoid Arthritis, Itching Fibromyalgia Jaundice, Pain, Headache, Ringworm, Cramps

Anti-carcinogenic, Anti-bacterial, Anti-inflammatory

Cautions:

Do not take medication those who suffer from Diabetes, GERD or Gall Bladder issues

* Do not take if you are taking anticoagulant medications.

* Do not take if you are you are suffering from a hormone disruption health condition.
* Do not consume when you are pregnant or nursing.
Avoid for 2 days prior and after surgery
* Could decrease the chances of men having a child.

Valerian
Anxiety, Depression, Insomnia and Convulsions. Epilepsy, ADHD, Stress, Headache, Mild Tremors, Muscular & Joint Pain, Fibromyalgia, Chronic Fatigue Syndrome, Menopausal Problems Upset Stomach
Cautions:
* It slows in the Central Nervous System so avoid for 2 weeks prior to or following surgery.
Small amounts of it can be okay during pregnancy and nursing, however it is recommended to stay clear of
* Avoid drinking alcohol when taking valerian.
Avoid taking sedatives , or any other medication that is influenced by the liver.

Yarrow

Gingivitis, Colds, Fever, Hay Fever, Diarrhoea
Stomach Upsets Flatulence, Bloating, Toothache
Cautions:
Avoid if you are breastfeeding or pregnant.
* Do not take while taking anticoagulants.
Avoid for two days prior and after surgery
* Do not apply if you are sensitive to any of the
plants within the family of ragweeds.
* Do not take if you are taking any medications
that contains lithium.

Chapter 8: Herbal Remedies For Children

There are a few easy to grow herbs that can make fantastic solutions for children. Children can also learn to cultivate their own remedies! Your children's herb garden should be based upon their age.

When you are in the yard, pick plants that have a vibrant color like calendula. Lamb's ears can be fuzzy and enjoyable for children as they're soft and may be used as bandsages to cover small scratchings. Children love to play with them. Children of older ages love learning that this is"the "toilet paper mill." Mullein is also known as the "toilet paper mill."

You can plant a variety of herbs that smell delicious and taste wonderful. Lemon balm, as well as other mints are always a favorite among children. It is good to know that these plants are easy to grow and can withstand even the tender attention of the most tender children.

Utilize your herb garden as an opportunity to

educate children about the natural world, prepare healthy meals, and create exciting art projects. The most effective herbal remedy for kids and all ages is to enjoy the herbs that are growing in the soil. An herb garden in front of the window could introduce children to the world of nature.

Here are a few of the top herbs for children. In addition, all of these herbs are also beneficial for adults.

Dill (Anethum Graveolens)
The most well-known flavoring ingredient used in making pickles. It's also a fantastic solution for children.

I got the biggest harvest of dill in the largest tub this year. It is one of the smaller varieties, which meant it didn't break and the seeds came in a steady stream!

Try squeezing the finely cut leaves and seed heads in between the Pages of an old telephone book to make homemade craft projects. It's simple and enjoyable.

In my practice, I utilize Dill as a great remedy for respiratory issues. It's extremely secure. Nursing mothers can consume an infusion of the leaves or make a decoction with the seeds to ease babies suffering from colic. The root can also be prepared however this is not something I've done. The seeds are useful and the leaves are delicious.

Incorporate dill into the bread recipe recipes. Rye bread is a staple. Dill also adds a fantastic flavor in stews.

Catnip (Nepeta Cataria)

Catnip may drive your cat mad however it's among the most effective herbs for relaxing and calm children. However, children aren't averse with cats , and don't think catnip is good for them. It has a peculiar bitter taste, and it is necessary to disguise the taste by using other herbs or create delicious preparations, such as syrup or sweets.

Catnip is my top choice to soothe discomfort from colic or teething. It's a great way to relax and is the perfect lukewarm bath for reduce a fever.

Catnip can help ease the symptoms of diarrhea during childhood. I use it in conjunction with blackberry leaves and dill to help with this problem.

If you are experiencing mild hyperactivity, you can mix catnip with lemon balm passionflower or chamomile.

Calendula (Calendula Officinalis)
Calendula is often referred to as 'pot marigold.' It's a flower that can be eaten. If you're able to grow your own calendula, be aware of how sticky they are. They're packed with Emollient healing substances that aid in the healing of wounds and also protect fragile skin.

My daughter makes an ointment using calendula flowers made with olive oil, and then spread it on her windowsill. She makes the fantastic balm to treat her baby's buttocks. Because of her exceptional treatment and this amazing cream, my daughter has never experienced an issue with her diaper. This is quite an achievement! It can be used to treat headaches, provided that there's no rupture in the eardrum.

Calendula's vibrant yellow and orange flowers are packed with skin-soothing benefits, phytochemicals, and nutrients that help cells heal themselves as well as fight the growth of fungal organisms and offer antiseptic protection against bacteria.

The herb is used to ease minor burns and shingles. In a hot poultice (or compress), it can lessen the discomfort of earaches.

It also helps reduce inflammation in the internal and external areas. It is utilized to heal ulcers, decrease fevers, and ease menstrual cramps and constipation.

Calendula when mixed with chamomile, creates an excellent hair rinse particularly suitable for hair that is blonde.

Making homemade remedies for children is fun, affordable and secure. Make sure to make remedies ahead of time so you can have ready in case your child experiences an "boo-boo" or is suffering from one of the most common childhood ailments.

Dollop of Dill, and Apple Lollipops
They are simple to prepare and great for stomachaches and loose stool. To ensure they are rich in vitamin C, you can add the rose hips with 2 tablespoons once you take the pan off the flame. Additionally, you can add 2 teaspoons of elderberries prior to warming the final juice to improve the immune system of your child.

Ingredients:
* Frozen pop molds
Two cups apple juice that is organic
* 2 teaspoons of dill seeds
Instructions:
1. The seeds can be crushed using a mortar and pestle . Or grind them into a coarse grind using the coffee grinder. In the juice 20 minutes, covered under low heat. Take the seeds off the stove.
2. Cool down. Then, filter then compost. The juice should be poured into molds made for soft drinks. Freeze until firm. The yield will vary based upon the amount of mussels.

Baby Bottom Balm

The baby shouldn't ever get diaper rash. Cleanse baby's skin after every diaper change, and give the skin to air out.

Apply a thin layer of this ointment in order to stop the urine and stool from irritating skin. It can also help in healing minor cuts and scrapes. Don't apply ointments to freshly burned areas; instead apply this after healing has begun.

Ingredients:
* 1 oz. calendula flowers
* 1 cup olive oil
* 2 tbsp. beeswax, grated
Instructions:
1. Put the herb in a pot that is clean. Cover them with oil. The oil will be able to cover the grass for approximately 1/8 inch. Blanket. Set it in a warm spot like an open window. Shake vigorously at minimum once per day. It should be left for two weeks.
2. The flowers should be filtered using an fine mesh strainer coffee filter, or cheesecloth and

add them to the compost pile. Be sure that all the elements of the plant are cleaned.

3. Combine the beeswax and oil in a double-boiler and stir until wax is melted. Stir. Continue heating for another minute. Pour the mixture into clean used baby jars, used baby jars as well as other containers. Cool. Cover the lids.

4. The yield is one cup. The ointment doesn't need to be refrigerated due to the beeswax.

Catnip Bath Fever Remedy

It's a great remedy for reducing fever. If your child suffers from an illness that causes irritation to the skin it is possible to place the oatmeal in two cups into an unclean sock or stocking and then add it into the tub to calm the skin of your child.

Ingredients:
• 1 cup catnip
Four cups of water that is boiling
Instructions:
1. Put boiling water in the bowl over catnip. Blanket. Sort the herbs and compost them.
2. Let the infusion of catnip cool until it reaches room temperature.
3. Include it in a warm bath (the bath shouldn't be cold or hot).

4. Your child can take a bath for at least 20 minutes.

Nature's Medicinal Balloons to Treat Ear Infections Flu, and other respiratory ailments
This recipe conceals the taste of the herbs with less flavor and has been traditionally used to treat fever and cure illnesses. I make it for my children when they are suffering from respiratory illness. They taste delicious and are packed with nutrients.

Ingredients:
1 cup almond butter
* 1/4 cup honey
* 2 tbsps. Echinacea root powdered
* 1 tbsp. catnip, powder
* 2 tbsps. elderberries dried and chopped
* 1 tbsp. rose hips Ground
Chocolate chips made from organic ingredients or raisins
* Coconut grated unsweetened
Instructions:
1. Mix all the ingredients together, except for the coconut. Mix well using your hands.
2. You'll find very firm and sweet candies.
3. Make balls that are that are the size of one

nickel using your hands. Then, roll them in coconut grated. Then, store the mixture in the refrigerator.

4. I recommend this candy be eaten 3-4 times throughout the daily. Below is my dosage chart that shows the amount to feed children of various age groups.

Dosage for Children's Age

Ages 3-5 1 ball for each dose

(3 or 4 times per each day)

6-11 years old. 1 whole ball to take a dose

(3 up to four times per every day)

12 years old or older 2 balls per dosage

(3 or 4 times per every day)

Be sure that they do not try to eat more because they're delicious and there's no need for more.

Constipation

Children may experience constipation from time to time. This is particularly common when they are experiencing an "difficult" eating stage and don't eat the right diet. This is the perfect opportunity to educate them about how important it is to get their bowels functioning properly.

Try this herbal recipe for a candy to help you relax.

Go Balls
Ingredients:
1 cup date (you could also use prunes or apricots)
1 cup of hot prune juice
1. 1/4 cup almond butter
* 1/8 cup flax seeds finely ground
* 1/4 cup of oatmeal.
Instructions:
1. Incubate the dates in the prune juice for 15 mins. Remove the juice and save the juice. Put the dates along with flax seeds, almond butter as well as half the oatmeal into the food processor. Process until you have a dough-like shape.
2. Add the remaining oats or juice in the amounts needed to create the consistency of a firm paste with a food processor and finally your hands. Form balls about that are the size of the size of a nickel using your hands.
3. Keep the candy in your refrigerator. Your child should eat this candy once or twice each day. Here is a dosage chart that will help you keep track of.

Dosage for Children's Age
3 to 5 years old 1 ball per dose
(1 to 2 times per each day)
6-11 years old 2 balls for each dose
(1 to 2 times per every day)
12 years and older 3balls plus for each dose
(1 to 2 times per each day)

Roll the balls into crushed nuts, if the child enjoys the idea, since nuts provide the fiber.

Stings, bites and Rashes
Insects seem to love the smell of soft skin and warm blood in young children. Did you notice that when there's poison oak or poison Ivy or poison sumac in the area, kids are bound to get their hands on it?

The affected area should be cleaned thoroughly with soap and water. Keep the paste in the hand to ease swelling and itching. The paste speed up drying of oozing rashes.

Anti-Itch clay for healing
Ingredients:
* 2 tbsp. peppermint leaf (you could replace 5 drops of essential oil, or 20 drops of tea oil from

trees)

* 1 cup of cosmetic clay (any kind will work children love vibrant clays, like green or orange)

13 cup Witch Hazel Extract

* 1 cup boiling water

Instructions:

1. Make a powerful drink by covering the peppermint leaves in boiling water.

2. Cover and let stand for 20 minutes.

3. After cooling when cool, separate the herbs from the liquid. The herbs should be firmly pressed against a colander in order to obtain every healing power from the mint. Then, discard the herbs. Save the tea.

4. Put the clay in an container that has a secure lid. Pour the witch hazel as well as herb tea in the clay, mixing continuously. Add the liquid until you have an even paste.

5. Cover the container with the protective cover. Make sure you label the container with a clear label by indicating that it's intended for use by the outside only.

6. If your children have grown older, and there's no way they'll consume the dough, put it in the refrigerator to keep it fresh. In other words keep it out of the reach of children at temperatures that are at room temperature.

7. Apply a cream or lotion to the skin when insects bite or rashes happen. (It can also help with hemorrhoids.) Wash after drying or as needed.

Chapter 9: Herbals To Treat Skin Problems

In many cases, our skin takes some punishment for the actions you do on it daily routine. The sun's rays and not applying enough lotion and even issues such as eczema can cause our skin to appear older and wrinkled than the years we've lived. There are a myriad of cosmetics available that claim to deliver the results you desire in clearing your skin and looking stunning, the majority of them do not work or contain additional ingredients that damage the skin. Herbs can be utilized to treat your skin in a natural and safe manner. There are a variety of plants that do an amazing job of caring for the skin, without drying out it or doing harm. No matter what's problem with your skin, or the things you want to see improve, the herbs can aid you.

The Best Herbs for Skin Care

Almond Oil

Almond oil is used to treat skin problems for a long time. It can help treat and even soften skin. Raw almond kernels offer gentle exfoliation that will remove dead skin cells. This will help to make your skin appear nice and clear in a matter of minutes. Additionally, almond oil is great for providing essential nutrients for the skin, which include vitamin A, protein, and minerals. It can be used on any type of skin and can help to ease itching, inflammation dryness, and itching. Alongside helping with your skin almond oil can be beneficial for lowering unhealthy cholesterol level, assisting people suffering from diabetes. It's one of the most effective ingredients for the face scrub as compared to regular soap for facials.

Geranium Oil

Geranium oil is used for many things apart from skincare and beauty, but it's great at giving the radiant glow you desire from your skin. It contains astringent properties which help clean and unblock pores to help you remove acne and help your skin appear clean and beautiful. Utilizing this product once per day or once every couple of days can make a significant impact on how beautiful your skin will appear.

Apart from giving your skin a glowing appearance, geranium oil can be great for relieving various other ailments that are common. It can help heal sore throats and cold sores wounds and infections. People have utilized geranium to alleviate the discomfort caused by an outbreak of shingles and may even help cure head lice.

Patchouli Oil

The next item on your list of herbal remedies for your skin are patchouli oils. There are occasions that your skin will begin to be extremely dry and itchy, maybe when the seasons begin to change, or you've used other products that don't work for your skin. Patchouli oil can be very beneficial to treat dry skin and help to hold in some moisture vital to the skin, and making your body and face appear ready for any challenge.

This is an oil that some people love but aren't so certain about, mainly because the smell is intense. If you're able to take the scent in your stride it is likely that Patchouli is excellent for the skin and is an effective herb to reduce depression and control your appetite.

St. John's Wort

If you're dealing with injured skin St. John's Wort is the solution you must take immediately. It can help heal any burns you suffer caused by sunburn or because you got too close to making meals in your kitchen. If your skin is damaged due to being outdoors or other activities in the daytime, St. John's Wort will aid you a lot.

Skin care is only one of the many uses for St.

John's Wort. Other benefits you can benefit from this herb are relieving depression and anxiety as well as helping people with incontinence, treating flu virus (although it's not very efficient with colds) and also helps to ease the muscles that are aching due to joints, arthritis, fibromyalgia and sciatica.

Witch Hazel

Witch hazel can be helpful with numerous issues on your skin. If you suffer from an in-sect burn, a bite, or scratches, witch hazel can be the plant which can help. It's also one of the primary treatments utilized for varicose veins as it is able to cleanse the area and reduce the pain during treatment.

There are a variety of other uses which you can get from witch hazel depending on your requirements. Many people prefer using witch hazel for acne combatant because it is effective by reducing swelling that is associated with blemishes and pimples. It acts as a toner, which helps to reduce the appearance of wrinkles and fine lines that show up on your face. Witch hazel works well for all skin types to reduce acne and prevent the effects of ageing on your skin and face.

Calendula Oil`

Calendula oil can be used for a variety of things to do with your skin. It's great for helping to heal your skin from any skin blemish or injury you might have. It doesn't matter if you're suffering from an injury or cut or you have minor cuts or insect bites. Calendula oil could be the answer to making your skin appear gorgeous. A lot of people have used this oil to aid in the case of acne, irritation to the skin and dry skin. With the anti-inflammatory as well as antibacterial properties of the oil, it could be used as a regular facial wash that makes your skin look more slack.

Your skin is among your most important assets. It's among the first things people will notice about you when you step out the door. Therefore, you need to ensure that your skin appears as glowing and beautiful like you. Make use of these plants and oils and notice how amazing your skin will appear in no time.

How to Care for Your Skin
Dry Skin
2 oz. almond oil
6 Tbsp. brown sugar
6 drops geranium oil
1 oz. honey
1. In a jar add the almond oil, honey as well as

brown sugar. Mix and mix. Then, add the geranium oil. Place the lid over.

2. Once you are ready the sugar will be at its highest and you can apply it to your skin.

3. Wash the mixture clean and then dry it before adding the moisturizing agent.

Eczema

1/4 c. olive oil

1/4 1 c. Oat flour

8 drops patchouli essential oil

1/2 1. coconut oil

Directions:

1. In the coconut oil, melt it until it's liquid, then adding the oat powder and the patchouli oil. Continue stirring thoroughly.

2. Incorporate the olive oil prior to taking off the stove and pouring the mix into an container.

3. Cool completely, then keep it in a tightly closed container.

4. Apply the cream to the region as needed, and then keep in a cool, dry place.

Cleaning and care for your nails and hands

2 drops of lavender oil

4 drops of chamomile oil

2 oz. olive oil

1 oz. grated beeswax

6 Tbsp. sugar

Directions:

1. Place the sugar in an jar that is small. Install an oven double boiler. Add an olive oil as well as beeswax. Stir them over at a low temperature to aid melt the beeswax. Remove off the heat and allow to let it cool.

2. Pour the beeswax as well as olive oil into the Jar and allow it to cool for five minutes. Mix in both the lavender and chamomile oils then put the cap on the top.

3. If you're ready After you're ready, massage a small amount of this onto your feet and hands for about a minute. Rinse off with warm water, and then relax!

Sunburn

16 drops St. John's wort oil

1 oz. calendula oil

7 oz. witch hazel

Directions:

1 .Pick one bottle with the cap that sprays. Mix the ingredients in it and shake thoroughly before making use of.

2. Once you are ready apply the spray to the area that is affected then allow the spray to soak into the skin prior to dressing.

Chapter 10: Home Remedies For Ligament, Joint, Tendons And Joint Conditions

Your ligaments, joints and tendon comprise soft tissues which permit you to move effortlessly. The muscles are the main mover in your body. The tendons of your bones connect to your muscles and aid in the transfer of forces across your joints to allow your skeletal system move. The ligaments that connect your bones. They are essential for the stabilization of your joints.

If you experience an issue with your soft tissues you could try using natural solutions. Ailments affecting ligaments, joints and tendons may range from mild to serious. The degree of pain, discoloration or swelling that you experience will depend on the extent of your injury. Note that minor injuries can be treated with the assistance of natural remedies. It is possible that you require medical attention when your injuries are serious. Based on Sharol Tilgner who is a naturopathic doctor and specialist on herbal medicines, issues that affect ligaments, joints muscles, and tendons can be addressed with herbal remedies which have anti-inflammatory and pain relieving properties. Devil's claw, for example is one of the most popular herbs to treat tendon, ligament and muscle issues. It can also be used combat back pain, arthritis, and other disorders that affect the gallbladder and kidneys as well as the liver. Phyllis Balch, a nutritional consultant and nutrition researcher says that this herb can be effective in relieving symptoms of soft tissue injuries like pain and inflammation. In addition to devil's claw there are many other herbs that have anti-inflammatory properties. A few of them include arnica as well as fennel, ashwagandha feverfew and gingko biloba. ginger, ginseng, licorice, and lavender.

To help ease the pain caused by soft tissues, pick from celandine, comfrey goldenrod, dong quai as well as myrrh, gotu kola as well as passionflower and the kava. If you're suffering from arthritis, you may make use of a range of herbs or plants that can treat your problem. Natural remedies can offer relief. Make sure to obtain a written approval from your physician prior to.

Aloe Vera can be helpful in the treatment of arthritis. You can purchase Aloe Vera gel to apply on painful joints. Boswellia is commonly referred to as frankincense is highly sought-after by many health professionals who use alternative therapies for the anti-inflammatory qualities it has. It is a blocker of leukotriene and other elements which affect joints in rheumatoid and other autoimmune disorders. It is available as a tablets or creams applied to the skin.

It is also possible to utilize Eucalyptus. The leaves of the plant contain tannins that can help to reduce pain and swelling. According to the National Center for Complementary and Alternative Medicine suggests ginger because it is anti-inflammatory and may reduce swelling in joints. The NCCAM also suggests green tea for its ability to decrease swelling and treat osteoarthritis.

4. Natural remedies to Eczema

Eczema is the term that is used to describe a variety of medical conditions that cause irritation or inflammation of the skin. It is identified by scaly, itchy patches. It is a problem that affects between 10 and percent of infants, and as high as three percent of adult patients across the United States. This is roughly 9.5 million individuals, which means you're not the only one. Children can outgrow the condition prior to adolescence, however most people experience signs and symptoms for the remainder of their lives. If you are suffering due to this condition there's no reason to be concerned as it's possible to control eczema by taking proper care. These natural treatments can ease the symptoms of eczema and enable you to identify any triggers that could increase the frequency of episodes. Like all changes to your regimen for skin care diet, lifestyle, and nutrition be sure to consult your primary physician prior to making any changes.

Coconut Oil

As coconut oil has became more widely used in the last year it is now more affordable and easier to obtain top-quality oil. Coconut oil is an excellent moisturizer, which soothes skin that is inflamed and provides relief from itching. It is also utilized in lieu for other essential oils used in natural, homemade exfoliants to rejuvenate and protect your skin. Coconut oil that is organic and virgin is the preferred choice because other ingredients can be added during processing. There are soaps and other skin care products that are made with coconut oil that may ease symptoms and aid in reducing future symptoms. Apart from being an excellent product for skin coconut oil can also be used in baking and cooking instead of more refined oils. It is free of hydrogenation, a process that transforms liquid fats to solid. It isn't a rich source of cholesterol like oils derived from animals.

Fatty Acids in Oils

Gamma-linolenic Acid (GLA) is an essential fatty acid which is extremely difficult to locate in our modern diets. GLA is an omega-6 fat acid which has been proven to decrease inflammation and growth of cells therefore it is logical that it could be beneficial in treating and management of eczema. It is found in the oils of plant seeds like borage oil, black currant oil as well as evening primrose oil and can be purchased in pills at the local health food retailer. Research has shown that GLA aids in nourishing hair, skin, as well as nails after 6-8 weeks after taking capsules.

Diet

It is now evident that diet and lifestyle aspects could be the main causes of Eczema. Some topical treatments may help reduce itching and reduce the appearance of the appearance of skin scaly, but most likely not resolve the root of the problem. Many people suffering from eczema are benefited by elimination diets, where any triggers, including wheat, dairy and soy are eliminated completely from the diet over a period of a month or more. It typically takes between two and four weeks for these foods to be eliminated from your body, allowing the body's system to reset. After that, you'll gradually introduce these foods back to see the foods to which your body is sensitive to based on whether you experience an allergic reaction.

Similar to diet changes Probiotics are a great option to improve the health of your stomach and intestines , as well as regulate the flora of your body. A lack of balance in the way your body digests and processing food could cause inflammation in your body which manifests itself in your eczema. These live organisms comprise that are essential to digestion, maintaining the immune system as well as the intake of nutrition. They are naturally found in fermented food items and are also present in soft cheeses and yogurt. If you're looking to introduce more probiotics in your diet through food such as yogurt, the label should read "live and active cultures" to reap the greatest benefits and optimal outcomes.

Chapter 11: Herbs For Curing Pain And Inflammation

Feverfew

This herb has been shown to be effective in curing and preventing migraines. Its active component in the herb works to lower the levels of serotonin in your body while relaxing the blood vessels that are located inside the brain. Other migraine-related symptoms that this herb is capable of treating are reducing nausea, vomiting, pain and heightened sensitivity to sound or light. It is particularly beneficial if you suffer frequently with migraines, in order to decrease the frequency of migraine attacks.

To achieve the desired result for the desired effects, take around 50-250 milligrams of dried feverfew leaves, which is equivalent to 3 fresh leaves as well as without. You can also prepare an tincture by dissolving the grinded leaves in alcohol. Its active components are the components parthenolide as well as tanetin. Both are the reason for the beneficial properties of feverfew for healing.

Witch Hazel

If you suffer from ailments such as hemorrhoids will benefit from the anti-inflammatory properties of this plant. Witch hazel offers numerous benefits , such as reducing itching and discomfort that comes with hemorrhoids. It also reduces the irritation and burning of the rectal area.

Witch hazel has active compounds like tannins and flavanoids, which can be volatile oil that help as a stopper of bleeding. Its bark has proven efficient to stop internal bleeding by injections into the rectum. This procedure is designed to decreasing the pain and itching that is caused by hemorrhoids. If you want to take care of your vagina it is possible to clean the area affected by applying pressure, wiping or bloating.

Chinese Skullcap

The herb is part of the mint family, and can be effective in reducing the symptoms of stress and headaches and insomnia, as well as premenstrual symptoms. Chinese skullcap is extremely efficient in combating arthritis-related inflammation. It is because of active ingredients like Baikal skullcap and catechu that are also known as flavocoxid. Other ailments that Chinese skullcap may treat include the inflammation of airways of the lung and bronchiolitis and various lung illnesses. The combination of Baikal skullcapand honeysuckle, and forsythia is effective in children who suffer from bronchiolitis. The disease is typically caused by respiratory syncytialvirus infection.

Meadowsweet

Meadowsweet is a source of active ingredients which are present in aspirin. Chewing the roots can aid in the reduction of headaches and other discomforts. The active components in this herb are salicylic acid and tannins. These are substances that your body readily converts into aspirin. Meadowsweet is especially beneficial when you have gastritis and arthritis, which is a condition that causes an inflammation of the stomach's lining.

The most effective way to consume the herb is by incorporating it into teas made of extracts of herbs. It is recommended that the amount of herb content is around 4 grams of meadowsweet to the herb. The tea can be made by adding 4-6 grams of dried herb, and consume the tea three times per day.

Chapter 12: Facial Scrubs

Based on the type of skin you have the best products for you are various ingredients.

Oily Skin

It's a complexion that occurs when two conditions are present:

1. Your skin produces more natural oils making your skin oily.

2. The skin may be dry, but it is trying to draw moisture from the air surrounding it, which is often what makes it oily.

The best method to regulate the production of oils by your skin in the event that your complexion is caused by the first issue is to monitor your diet and record your meals you've had. There are certain foods that you can consume that make your skin produce oil.

If you avoid these foods and foods, you will be able to control the production of oil on your skin. Additionally, you should ensure that the cleanser you use don't dry your skin. This could make oily skin appear worse.

The second issue is quickly identified. After cleansing your skin, measure how long it takes for your skin to change from oily to dry. If it takes around an hour or so before you begin to notice the appearance of a sheen, then you might be suffering from the second issue.

Wash your face at least at least once per day, and allow your face to dry. Then, follow this with an oil-based moisturizer to keep the face soft and silky. If you wash your face at least once per day isn't going to send your skin go into overdrive with regard to the natural oils your body produces by itself.

Extra Ingredients for Oily Skin

There are a few things you can include to your

scrub to aid in the absorption of the oils that are left:

Oatmeal

Finely ground oatmeal is recognized, not just to help absorb oil however, it also helps keep skin smooth.

Clay powders

The addition of a small amount the powder to a scrub will aid in absorbing oils on the skin.

Skin Scrub Oily I

12 Cup brown sugar
1 tbsp Ground peppermint
1/2 1 tbsp ground oatmeal
3 Tbsp Sweet Almond Oil
2 drops Clary Sage
4 Drops Petitgrain
4 Drops Ylang Ylang
2 Drops of Peppermint

Face Scrub II Oily Face Scrub II

12 Cup Sea Salt
1 Tbsp Ground Calendula Petals
1/2 tbsp ground clay powder
3 Tbsp Sweet Almond Oil
2 Drops Altas Cedarwood
4 Drops of Carrot Seed
4 . Drops of Tea Tree
2 Drops Myrrh

Dry Skin

The type of skin can vary from a mild ashy look to eczema or the psoriasis. There are several actions you can take to manage the appearance of your dry skin.

1. Apply a moisturizer to your skin every morning and prior to going to go to bed.

2. Take moisturizer along in your makeup kit , ready to apply as needed.

3. Let your skin air dry. Your skin will then soak of the moisture naturally.

4. Cleanse your face with warm water. Hot water can dry your skin.

Sometimes, eczema or Psoriasis is the cause from an allergic response to food or an environmental ingredient. See a doctor who can provide you with an allergy test to identify the food or substance that could be the cause of the rashes.

Dehydration may result in your skin drying and become ashy or even begin to crack. To determine if your skin is dehydrated, place a tiny amount of your skin on the surface of your hand, and then release it.

When the skin is snapped instantly to its original position You're fine. If your skin is slowly moving back to its original position it is important to drink water. Consuming coconut water, drinking liquid, or any other non-alcoholic drink, such as juice, will provide your body the water it requires to continue its journey.

Avoid using the scrubs on broken or cracked skin.

Extra ingredients for dry skin

Two herbs could add to your arsenal of herbs to assist in battling dry and flaky skin.

Kelp

This herb is rich in minerals and vitamins that your skin requires to stay healthy and heal.

Horsetail

Another herb will enhance the effect of the scrub, and help soften skin.

Dry Skin Scrub

12 Cup Brown Sugar
1/2 Tbsp Kelp
1/2 Tbsp Horsetail
1 Tbsp Sweet Almond oil
1 Tbsp Coconut oil

6 Drops Lavender

4 Drops Patchouli

2 Drops Geranium

Dry Scrub for Face II

1/4 Cup Brown Sugar

1/8 Cup Sea Salt

1 2 tablespoons Kelp

2 tablespoons coconut oil

4 Drops Ylang Ylang

4 Drops Rose

2 Drops of Frankincense

2 Drops of Carrot Seed

Normal Skin

Normal skin requires care and love, too We
haven't forgotten about it.

If you have a regular routine that is working for you and you are sticking to it, continue it. A typical routine could appear like:

Wash face before getting up in the morning.
Moisturize following washing.
Three times a week.
Nightly moisturizing
Light washing after removal of make-up

Regular Maintenance I

12 Cup Brown Sugar
3 Tbsp Sweet Almond Oil
4 Drops Ylang Ylang
4 Drops Lavender
4 Drops of Peppermint
3 Drops of Carrot Seed
3 Drops Chamomile

Regular Maintenance II

12 Cup Brown Sugar
3 Tbsp Sweet Almond Oil
4 Drops Chamomile
4 Drops Rose
4 Drops Ylang Ylang

3 Drops Geranium

3 Drops Lavender

Chapter 13: Headache And Fever Solutions

Today, taking pills to ease headaches has become so popular that people don't even is aware of the potential side effects it may be causing. We can safely say that yes, there are certain negative side effects that occur in the course of use. It isn't necessary to resort to synthetic remedies to eliminate headaches, however. There are many natural remedies can be used to relieve the throbbing pain that is associated with these aches. If you're experiencing headaches following your work take a look at one of these remedies: Ginger tea - It's been used in Asia for thousands of years in place of aspirins. All you have be able to crush approximately 1 inch of ginger and then add the crushed ginger to boiling water. It will help to decrease inflammation and take about similar time to aspirin to be effective.

Capsaicin cream can be prepared at home or bought from a health store. The active ingredient is cayenne pepper. To use it, you'll have to place a small amount in your nostril on the side of your head that the pain is. What exactly does it do? The cream blocks pain signaling from nerves, thereby considerably reducing discomfort.

Feverfew - In numerous clinical studies, it has been found that this ingredient of the sunflower family can be extremely powerful in treating the most dreadful migraine. It assists reduce inflammation, which removes any pressure of the nerves . It could even completely stop migraines.

Mint Juice Mint is antiseptic as well as anti-pruritic qualities that can be beneficial in relieving headaches. Menthone and menthol both are excellent for this in addition to. To make use of it you can put mint tea compresses placed on your forehead to ease any discomfort. You may also apply mint juice along with your temples for a more effective treatment. In addition to mint juice, you could also try one composed of coriander.

Lavender Oil The benefits of lavender are well-known. Do you realize that lavender could also be used to treat headaches? It's easy all you need to do is mix lavender oil to an ice-cold bow and then inhale the vapors that come out of it. You can do this for a couple of minutes each day or as often as you require it. You may also apply it externally on the forehead while massaging your temples. Be sure to never inhale lavender oil by mouth.

After having some basic headache cures
discussed, what do we do about the most
dreaded fever? Most of the time, similar to
headaches, many people will take prescription
medications to treat it. Yes, it is effective but
there are more natural and safe remedies are a
good option to try when you're feeling unwell.
Here are some suggestions:

Chamomile tea is among the most sought-after
kinds of tea that is more than just able to bring a
sense of peace and calm for people. It is also a
great option to reduce a person's fever.
Additionally, it's also able to treat muscles pain,
cramps and anxiety.

Echinacea was used over the centuries by Native
Americans when it comes to treating colds and
influenza. This herb can aid in strengthening the
immune system, making us less prone to illness as
well as reduce the chance of your fever returning.

Gingkgo is also called ginkgo biloba this well-
known herb is known as a treatment for fevers. In
addition, it is well-known for its effectiveness in
enhancing the brain's activity as well as blood
circulation. It's offered in tea form, making it easy
to consume. Consume it every day in conjunction
with meals.

St. John's Wort - A popular alternative to

prescription depression medications and can also lower fevers and strengthen the immune system as it is used to treat the body.

Chapter 14: Superior Beverages Options

Are you a victim of the power of caffeine? Are you among the people who have already spent hundreds of dollars for energy drinks? Perhaps you're allergic (or any other stimulant) which is why you're searching for a different option. Whatever your reasons is we'll help you discover 25 great ways to combat fatigue.

The first is to sip a glass of cool water. It's fine if you're slightly sceptical about this idea, however. In the end, it may appear to be too easy to offer any real benefits. However, keep in mind that cold temperatures cause blood-rushing that occurs when cold water moves through your body, the whole circulatory system accelerates the key functions.

What happens when blood flow increases (particularly towards important organs)? The body goes into an alert state (since it's shielding it from the abrupt drop in temperature) and this implies that the mind will instantly be free of any thoughts that is related to sleeping. If you're truly feeling exhausted you may want to consider a strategy that relies on sugar.

As you'd expect The second method of fighting fatigue is drinking a sugar and water solution. You're probably thinking about one concern - aren't you thinking that sugar is a stimulant similar to caffeine? In reality, it isn't. A lot of people assume it is. In the end, children who consume sweets in a jiffy can are prone to all kinds of trouble (in other words, they go through periods of high-activity).

What is the role of sugar in boosting alertness? There are two ways to answer that. The first concern sugar's high energy content and its structure's simplicity. That is, whenever you consume a concoction of sugar and water the body will experience an immediate boost in energy because it doesn't require the processing of sugar in the same manner as other substances that increase vigor.

Apart from providing calories to burn, a sugar and water beverage can also increase the amount of insulin that your body produces. For a better explanation when the body senses that sugar levels are rising the body produces more insulin , so that sugar levels will drop in a short time. Insulin is a beneficial "side effect" however - when it becomes more abundant it causes the brain to end up being stimulated.

If you're not interested in drinking sugar-free water, you may prefer this energy booster mixing lemon juice (or some slices of fruit) to an ice-cold glass. Lemon juice, no matter the degree of sourness has sugar. It's not the same as table sugar it is, in particular because the sugar in fruit (which experts refer to as fructose) isn't a common ingredient to speed up the production of insulin.

Even though lemon water does provide the body with additional energy, it doesn't have as much calories as its table-sugar-containing counterpart. So, is adding some fruit juice to H2O an ineffective (but an easier for those with diabetes) option to mix water and sugar together? No, it's not. Lemon has a distinct sour taste that makes it a powerful energy booster.

After reading this you may think that drinking lemons with a sour taste water is an effective method of fighting insomnia. It could be a great option occasionally but don't make it into a routine. If you're wondering whythis is happening, take this in mind: any sour food can result in an increase in susceptibility to gastritis and can also cause the pain associated with ulcers.

Are there any drinks that are suitable for those

who don't drink cold water, but suffers from diabetes as well as stomach problems? There is a solution the answer - soymilk. It's important to mention immediately, however, that this vegan substitute of fresh milk from cows is a source of some purine in small amounts - an ingredient that is linked to both joint and insulin issues.

It wouldn't be a good idea to consume an entire glass of soymilk every when you're feeling exhausted. Consuming just one glass a every day is sufficient in the event of a medical issue that is related to uric acids. If you're in good health and aren't getting many purines from the rest in your food, 2 to three glasses are sufficient.

Although you're aware that soymilk isn't something you can drink throughout your entire day, you aren't sure how to eliminate the fatigue feeling. The abundance of Vitamin B12 makes the beverage an ideal alternative to stimulant-rich drinks. Sleepiness can be an indication that you have a Vitamin B12 deficiency.

Do you know of a substitute for soymilk that tastes a little better? The lemon water itself doesn't taste like lemon water, does it? If you were to include fruits in a regular shake of protein, then you'd be able to get something that has both high energy carbohydrates as well as B

Vitamins. Because the type of fruit you'd include will depend on your preference and preferences, there won't be any issues with flavor.

What you should be aware of: you shouldn't ignore the extra. Even if you're brave enough to drink a non-flavored shakes of protein (or you just need a less calorific drink) It's still necessary to add a few pieces of fruit in order that the B vitamins you'll get are helpful. In the end, these nutrients are the ones that speed up the process of converting food into energy.

Just to help you even further, here are several suggestions on which fruits could make your energy-booting beverage much more potent - strawberry (this fruit isn't merely good for the eyes, it's also rich in metabolism-accelerating Vitamin C), banana (a superb, nutritionally-diverse choice for people with digestive issues), and blueberry (known to enhance both mental focus and memory).

Chapter 15: Utilizing Natural Supplements To Cure Insomnia

It's tempting to use sleeping aids that are available over-the-counter or prescribed in the event of episodes of insomnia. The sleeping pills are not able to address the root cause of the issue. However, certain sleeping aids may cause you to have more insomnia over the long term. Before you decide to take any sleep aid, speak with your physician or pharmacist.

Many herbal and nutritional supplements are designed specifically to aid in sleep. Some of these treatments include lavender and chamomile tea , are, in the majority of cases safe. Other remedies may cause adverse effects that can cause problems with specific medications.

Lavender is a Lavender is a herb used to aid in the treatment of insomnia. The flower or oil from the lavender plant emit the scent of relaxation. There are many ways to use lavender, such as on the market in essential oil, scrub or bath additive, or a sachet , which can be put under your pillow.

Chamomile Tea - A cup of hot the tea before sleep is believed to aid people sleep. Make a cup of tea and relax as you wind down from your day.

Melatonin The hormone Melatonin is an hormone your body naturally produces at the night. It aids in regulating the cycle of sleep and wake. Melatonin supplements are effective in short-term usage. Many people utilize melatonin to reduce or prevent jet lag. A smaller amount of melatonin could be administered on a regularly basis with no negative consequences. Possible side effects from Melatonin usage could be an increase in drowsiness later on. You should take between 1 and 20 milligrams for 30 minutes prior to going to sleep. Even tiny doses of melatonin are proved to be efficient.

Valerian is a Valerian is a herb that has moderate sedative effects. The supplement could help you rest better. You can take between 400-900 milligrams valerian for up to two hours prior to going to sleep.

Hops - They are typically used to stabilize and as a flavoring agent for beer. It has been proven to ease the effects of insomnia. Hops as well as Valerian are very similar in appearance and both can have an sedative effect on individuals. Hops and Valerian are frequently used together to create an even stronger effect. A combination of 120 milligrams hops extract could to improve the quality of your sleep.

Magnesium and Calcium - A absence of these two nutrients could cause insomnia as well as the capacity to fall to sleep when awoken at the beginning at night. Every day, you must get 1,000 milligrams of calcium and approximately 350 milligrams magnesium.

If you're experiencing the effects of insomnia , and exhausted energy because of sleeping less There are some natural solutions you can take to fight the consequences of not getting an adequate night's rest. It is not the same as sleeping however, these supplements could help you get the extra boost you need when you are feeling tired.

Other than these herbs and salts There are other natural remedies that have been utilized to treat insomnia for many millennia. It is possible to combine them and testing their effectiveness to help you fall asleep, however it's not advised without consulting a medical professional first. Natural and herbal don't necessarily mean that they're safe for you, particularly since the majority of pharmacological medicines are made or obtained from natural materials. However, treatments such as Ashwagandha (increases endurance and reduces stress) and the ginseng (enhances cognitive sharpness) as well as cordyceps (reduces fatigue) and coenzymeQ10 (internal the production of energy) have been proven to be effective in treating insomnia.

These herbs can be found and other supplements at the neighborhood health store, or at a pharmacy. Like any medication or supplement, it is recommended that you should consult with your doctor prior to making use of it.

Chapter 16: Medicinal Herbs And Essential Oils

A major issues that we have to face is assumption in the notion that health care is a "one fit all' type of procedure. But of course, if we consider this for a moment of course, doctors practice medicine frequently
often tweak the treatment prior to getting the desired results.
Although we seem to accept this as normal however, we are quickly discouraged when our whole-person approach is not working.
choices perform disappointingly. What is the reason? What is the reason we allow some flexibility to a handful of aspects of our lives? and not any of the mystifications of Mother Nature?

Expectations
We believe in God's work is flawless however, we must remember that when we are using essential oils, herbs flowers, essential oils, and
These seem to falter and we are quickly disenchanted and the word that is most important"quickly. If we are able to do this,

In the beginning of the age of information and we were quickly taught. The patience of our children grew shorter
as our expectations continued to go beyond our imaginations. We let little ume to be used for
Anything, yet we want instantaneity from the way our body reacts to any kind of health.
Wellness treatment. If there isn't a noticeable reaction within a brief time frame the treatment off.
focus on another thing, becoming increasingly dissatisfied, and then and resigned.
In this regard the most effective solution is to reorient our thinking, and to understand the body is extremely adept at performing what it is required to accomplish. It's all it takes is the right time. When we expect immediate
is a result of organic or natural remedies result from natural or organic remedies. We are not allowing for an organic process. Look at the messages we transmit to our body through such ideas as these. But, on the other hand you can trust the
process, and giving the body the chance to absorb the treatments as it was created to do. are
The blessing of God's favor is the growth of health.

The Placebo Effect

The efficacy of any treatment or supplement will directly correlate with an individual's incongruity. A lot of people claim to integrate whole-body health practices into their routine however, there is a huge gap in the evidence. even go as that they invest lots of money and time in integrative techniques as well as plants-based

treatments, but do not adhere to the idea that any other alternative to western medicine is effective.

They can decide to give it a go as it appears to be it's the right thing to do or join an entire family

A friend or a member's suggestion and expressing appreciation for the issue; but, still not convinced of any

"New age" treatments will have an impact. In other words, you will feel the placebo effect, and They get what they expected.

You can give a person the sugar pill and inform them that it's a drug that promises to ease their nerves.

If they wish to be relaxed enough and feel relaxed, this is what they will experience. Tell someone

A essential oil can alleviate their pain, and even if the person thinks it's quackery the pain will go away.
remains. So, for any other holistic or western approach to be effective, the belief must be in alignment
after the procedure. Otherwise the patient is not experiencing a sense of
hopeless. To counteract this feeling, one must rethink his or her faith in God.
The perfection of God's work the perfection of God's work and Nature.

Bio Individuality
As human beings, no everyone is made the same or identical up right down to fingerprints.
We still believe that our bodies will respond to treatment and medications as our best friend or co-workers did. Because there are different genetics, environment such as diets, beliefs, and so on.
We're doing ourselves a disservice by limiting the scope of illness down to the prescribed approach. When working within a certain framework is certainly a good base
where to start and abide by the protocol, but failing to consider the more complicated

personal character is sure to erode the score. This is the place where a amount of sanity can creep into

The healthcare system for healthcare. The same procedure is tried repeatedly with different outcomes. If we

We really want to see positive results, we need to pay attention to the body! In

in other words, if a body doesn't respond positively within a reasonable time,

Then, tweaking the method and tweaking the method. This is requires a trained professional can be beneficial.

Highly highly. The person who is monitoring responses and give sensible suggestions.

The power of plants is immense and are effective to treat the human body. But, they can be a challenge in difficult situations or

When working synergistically with western medicines, and having the assistance of a herbalist,

Naturopath, Drugless Practitioner, etc. ensures safety and successful. Like other

medications, but they are not recommended under certain circumstances. This means that not only an individual's

Body chemistry plays a role in the effectiveness

equation, and so will the current drink of pharmaceuticals.

Medical practice, dental practice, massage practice, yoga practice; life takes practice. In reality,
throughout our lives regardless of how much training we receive in life, the only thing we can count on as we go through life is
change. Our bodies alter on an physical and on a cellular level year to year
from month to month and week to week as well as day-to-day. The factors that affect these variations are as subtle as the manner in which they occur.

We move, think, or consume food. For as complicated as our lives can be, any deviation from our natural inclinations generally goes
It was not noticed up to...

But, knowing this natural process allows us to position ourselves to build a stronger partnership with
the body. This awareness alters our expectations and gives us control over the results , and aids us by assisting in ensuring that the outcome with assisting the outcome to with assisting the outcome to be the best it can. We can all help in ensuring that the outcome will emerge from this

alive.

however, being a whole participant is about eliminating those things that do not work, in order for our body can function properly.

can be done as well as it is.

Chapter 17: Green And Red Tea

Although this article is titled green and red teas however, the other three colours that tea comes in are also covered to give you a better understanding of the benefits that different varieties of tea provide. Red and green are the two teas that are readily available and provide the greatest beneficial health benefits. This is why they are included under the heading.

Tea

The facts and figures regarding tea are far too numerous to cover in a single section of a book. However, this book will attempt to explain the basics of different kinds of tea, their qualities and health benefits that result from them, as well as an overview of the background.

Tea has been consumed for hundreds of years, and is one of the most commonly consumed beverages in the world.

The tea plant known as Camellia Sinensis as well as all kinds of tea (except red, as discussed below) originate from this. What differentiates each variety in terms of taste, colour, and nutritional value is determined by the time it is harvested and what processes it goes through. There are more than 3,000 kinds of tea, each having different characteristics.

Tea comes in five fundamental colors. The black tea that most people are familiar with, is green tea that is gaining popularity, the red tea of South Africa, also growing in popularity, though less quickly, and at present, under-appreciated white tea. Also, there is yellow tea, however it isn't yet available in many countries. Fruit and herbal teas aren't thought of as "real tea" and therefore are not element in this piece. Teas like red, Rooibos can also be classified as a herbal tea since it is derived out of the South African plant Aspalathus Linearis however, as tomatoes are considered vegetables when they're actually fruit and red tea is utilized as a normal tea.

Although China is the birthplace of tea Indian tea has become more extensively consumed. China Tea generally has a more robust flavour that takes time to get used to, whereas Indian Tea, which is lighter in taste and is less abrasive than other varieties is a favorite among a larger segment of the population. While it is a native of Asia The tea plant is grown across many countries, and each has their own unique flavour of tea. There are many brands of tea bags that contain Indian tea, whether Assam or Darjeeling So if you purchase a black generic tea bag or tea, the most likely it's Indian.

The History of Tea

There are many stories of how tea came to being a drink others say that while boiling water to sterilize it certain leaves fell into it It tasted great and that's how tea was born.

Tea is a plant that has been used in China for hundreds of years. It is not known the length of time this has been aroundfor, however, it is believed to be more than 3000 years old.

There is evidence of tea being consumed for medicinal purposes in the Han Dynasty (206 BCE-220 CE) in China and also as a basic drink between the 618-907 CE in the Tang Dynasty.

Tea leaves dried in the air were shipped to Europe during the 16th century, and this was the beginning of the tea phenomenon. Tea was expensive in the 16th century and only the nobility or the very wealthy could afford it and often they kept it in the tea caddy. These were intricate canisters. The initial ones resembled ginger jars, but eventually they changed to wooden containers with locks. This was to make sure only precise doses of tea were given to the owners and that nothing was stolen or wasted, since it was costly. When the cost of tea dropped also did the demand for tea chests, tea jars and caddies.

In addition to being a medicine as well as a normal drink tea has been and is still, utilized as a social event , like tea parties, afternoon tea There are important tea ceremonies across diverse cultures like those by Japan or China.

How Tea is Made

Tea leaves begin to lose their elasticity and then begin to oxidize after being picked. In this process, the leaves darken as chlorophyll (the green pigment in plants) as well as it releases tannins*.

The scientific term used to describe this is fermentation. the process is halted with heat, which inhibits the enzymes responsible for this reaction.

In the case of black tea, the heat is applied in the same manner as the leaves are dried.

Tea is typically classed based on the method used to make it and then processed.

The sequence is: the tea is picked, wilted, or the

tea is oxidized and crushed or bruised (black tea) Some type of heat-applied (steam baking, steaming etc., based on the tea being produced) then shaped and then dried.

*Tannins are naturally occurring polyphenols in plants. They are the component that gives the tart or bitter flavor to unripe fruits. Polyphenols and phenols that are natural are found in tea, and studies have shown that a particular group of flavonoids that could have benefits for health. Tannins are currently being researched since for a long time they were believed to be a little harmful, but more research suggests that certain tannins can be beneficial.

Making an Cup of Tea
Naturally, you add hot water to the tea, and then wait for it to cool before you take a sip. Everyone who drinks tea knows this. There are additional factors that tea drinkers who are serious consider essential for making tea properly and these are temperature and the time for steeping, as illustrated in the guide:
Black tea 99C for 2 to 3 minutes
Green tea 80C for 1 2 minutes
White tea 65C for 1 - 2 minutes
Tea in yellow - 70C for 1 to 2 minutes

The red tea is 95C over 1 minute

It is important to note that the temperature of water as well as time for steeping can affect the flavor dramatically, according to experts.

It is also crucial to heat the pot prior to making tea, as this permits the water to come in contact with the tea at the right temperature. The colder the pot, the more it cools down the water, however in a practical sense it also keeps your tea warm to enjoy.

Different Tea Colours and the benefits

In essence, all colours are the same tea (except red) The difference is that they are taken at various stages of the process and then dried or processed in various methods. There are a variety of tea that come in all colors However, the following is just a basic overview of the most common tea.

Black Tea

The most popular cup of tea, black tea and up until recently, it was the only kind offered in many countries. It's the one that's popular and any request for tea bags or tea leaves usually yields this kind.

It is typically split between Indian tea as well as China tea (why it is often referred to as China tea, and it is not Chinese tea, I was not able to find out.)

The more tea refined, less benefit can be derived from it. This is evident since the darker the shade the more work it has gone through. It is because black tea is the same as white tea, only in smaller amounts, however, in general it has advantages. The biggest variation is in antioxidant qualities, with the lighter teas possessing significantly more. While green tea contains around 30 percent of the caffeine content in the coffee cup and black tea contains about 50%, so although black tea contains higher levels of caffeine than the other varieties, it's nevertheless less than coffee.

M.B. Red tea is naturally caffeine-free.

Oolong is usually considered to be a different category as well however, since the tea is black it is included in the section on all teas that are black.

Green Tea

As with most teas, green tea was developed in China but due to the increase in the popularity of green tea, several other countries have begun expanding their production. The process of making and growing tea is different from one country to the next and that can result in different flavors and health benefits.

The results of research and the findings on the benefits of green tea for you have been found to be inconclusive.

This could be because of a variety of causes that aren't fully clarified:

Green tea tests were halted before the right number of tests were completed in order to establish as factual the health benefits when tests revealed positive results for all participants.

The results aren't available to the public , which makes you wonder why they even bother making any.

It's previously been studied on animal models and has amazing results, but it has never been tested on humans. It reduces cholesterol levels in animals (do the animals have high cholesterol?) So why not try this on people? There are no adverse side consequences to the consumption of green tea therefore there's no risk and surely lots to gain?

Green tea is a rich source of minerals, including manganese, selenium, zinc and chromium, as well as Vitamin C. It only contains 30 percent of the caffeine that is found in coffee.

Since there aren't any conclusive studies, this are

a few what green tea could do to help:
Cancer, heart disease kidney stones and cholesterol oral and dental hygiene bone density, insulin sensitivity and glucose tolerance brain function and fat metabolism body fat and weight assist in the protection of brain cells during cases of Parkinson's disease, Alzheimer's disease, and eye diseases.

White Tea
The tea white is made mostly by China it is made up of buds or young leaves that after drying, turn silver in colour. It is less processed than other teas and isn't oxidized, but it is allowed to wither and is quickly dried. It's similar to green tea, only little more sweet.
Research is not yet complete however, it is believed to be more effective in fighting cancer than tea. It can reduce the growth of viruses and bacteria and strengthen the immune system. Research suggests that white tea is an antioxidant and anti-inflammatory. It also has components that could reduce the risk of developing heart arthritis and rheumatoid arthritis but , as with different teas "more tests must be carried out before findings are conclusive". There's no mention of when these tests will be completed

however, as the study appears to be overdue it is likely that tests are not being reviewed.

Yellow Tea

Yellow tea is very scarce and can be difficult to locate. Similar as green tea, it's dried more slowly , making tea leaves yellow. The taste is between white tea and green tea, and is moderate. The color is more of an amber-colored hue rather than yellow, however it can vary from one brand to the next.

Red Tea

The term red tea is commonly used to refer to Rooibos which is which is Afrikaans meaning Red Bush as this is not just the most well-known tea in South Africa, but also the only tea that has been exported in a large way.

It's full of healthy components, such as minerals, vitamins, as well as the high levels of iron antioxidants, anti-spasmodic (help digestion issues) however it contains the least amount of caffeine and very little tannin. Even though it does not contain caffeine, it is not advertised as being de-caffeinated. This isn't de-caffeinated since it doesn't contain caffeine at all.

The process of eliminating caffeine typically

involves an approach that some experts believe isn't healthful, (although some say it's healthy) however, many authorities do believe that de-caffeinated beverages like tea and coffee are not truly caffeine-free.

A particularly excellent Rooibos is the tea that is smoked, and is distinctive and has an earthy taste.

Rooibos is a rich source of antioxidants. It also has no caffeine and has low tannin levels. Like green tea, studies aren't conclusive yet for various reasons that are difficult to comprehend However, it is believed it could aid in treating allergies, cancer and digestive disorders, nervous tension and asthma, to mention only few.

It is not known if there are adverse negative effects from drinking red tea.

(My favorite Red Tea I like to drink is Red Bush which has a fantastic smoky taste.)

There's an alternative South African Honeybush tea, close to Rooibos however, it is hard to locate in other parts of South Africa.

Fir Tree Tea

Though it's not something that you can purchase the tea you like, it's loaded with Vitamin C. beta carotene. Antioxidants, and I mean full!

It is made of pine as well as spruce, fir or cedar. Cut off the branches with six or seven at the end of the bud, around 4 inches in length, and boil the water for 2 to 3 minutes. Take it off and drink. It is delicious but slightly bitter. If you prefer sweet tea, include honey or the syrup of agave.

It's a great way to the most use out of to your tree for Christmas.

Conclusion

In the end tea, whether it's white, red green, black or white, seems to offer an aid or cure for various health issues - however, the "experts" haven't concluded tests that yield reliable results. Therefore, it is impossible to claim this and nothing seems to be being done on the scientific front to determine what tea actually can do. Perhaps it can replace medicines for a variety of health issues However, that could be a problem for the pharmaceutical industry, but who is aware of this.

Of all the claims about health that are made, even if they're not verified, none of them can be proven to be true. Tea is a nutritious, delicious drink, so enjoy it to relax, or take it to reap the its health advantages, however, continue drinking the pills at least for the moment.

Part 2. 10 NATURAL RESOURCES to halt the

growth of inflammations

1. Garlic

Every food has a distinct flavor due to the garlic. It's common knowledge that this potent spice can be effective in curing various illnesses. The most popular uses of garlic is as an anti-inflammatory. Garlic is beneficial in relieving swelling and pain in joints due to arthritis.

2. Black Pepper

Black pepper is often referred to in the sense of"the "king of the spices" and is full of aroma and flavors. Also, it has intoxicating qualities and is a source of piperine, which is a powerful anti-inflammatory drug. Piperine aids in the reduction of pain due to arthritis. It also helps to stop the spread of cancer.

3. Chamomile

Chamomile isn't just drinks that are soothing It also assists to reduce inflammation in the mouth. In particular, the oils produced by the chamomile flower have anti-inflammatory and antispasmodic qualities.

4. Ginger

If there is an award of popularity for traditional medicine, ginger is a certain winner. This is a proven remedy that has stood the test of time and is remains a popular treatment for common inflammation diseases. Additionally, it can be a great treatment for nausea, stomach upset vomiting and many other ailments.

5. Aloe

Aloe has been shown to be efficient in reducing inflammation and reduces pain associated with inflammatory conditions. It's often called "the beautifying plant" because of its ability to heal skin damage and regeneration or healing.

6. Pomegranate

It's a kind of antioxidant called flavonols which are efficient in the reduction of inflammation that is caused by osteoarthritis or the same type of disease. Additionally, it blocks the production of cartilage damaging enzymes.

7. Soy

Soy is rich in isoflavones. These can reduce inflammation and preventing its negative impact on damaging bones and joints. However, processing and preservation of soy should be avoided as much as is feasible.

8. Cayenne
Capsaicin is a component of cayenne peppers that is commonly employed as a component in creams and lotions that are applied topically to reduce pain and inflammation. However, doctors have warned that certain types of peppers may cause inflammation in people with Rheumatoid arthritis. Having advised that you determine what works best for you.

9. Tomatoes
The lycopene content of tomatoes is high which is a powerful anti-inflammatory. It can be consumed in the form of a juice or eaten raw and the best thing about tomatoes is that it creates more lycopene after cooking. It's an effective treatment for lung inflammations , among other.

10. Beets
Beets are also a fantastic sources of antioxidants. It can help reduce inflammation and pain. Beets

are also contains vitamin C as well as fiber and betalains that are powerful cancer fighting agents.

Chapter 18: Supplements And Herbs For Hypertension

Since the beginning of time, herbs have been employed to treat an variety of alignments and with reasons that are valid. Herbs can be a healthier alternative to medicines that cause severe side effects, and frequently perform better than prescribed counterparts. The following supplements and herbs are proven to be beneficial to those who suffer from hypertension.

Hawthorn

Hawthorn is a herb that must be stored in any heart health medicine chest. It is high in flavonoids that can aid in reducing heart problems such as palpitations, blood pressure and arrhythmia. It has also been shown to be beneficial in controlling glucose metabolism and improving the function of the capillaries. It can be used in many forms, like tea or"balls". The hawthorn herbal"balls"recipe comprises cinnamon and ginger and cinnamon, two useful ingredients that help to improve circulation. For this recipe, you'll require:

* 4 tablespoons hawthornberry Powdered

* 1/2 to 1 tablespoon ground cinnamon
* Raw honey
* Water
* Carob powder , or cocoa powder

In order to make herbal ball make the balls, mix ground cinnamon and the powdered hawthorn berry in the bowl. Add the honey and just enough water to mix until it turns into a paste. Add carob powder and cocoa powder so that the mixture gets thicker and you can make dough balls. The mixture is then rolled into balls which are about the same size as your fingernail. Place the balls on a cookie sheet , and let them dry out in an oven that is set at 150 degrees. When the herbs are dry, place them in the glass jar.

Garlic

Garlic is a common home remedy food item that's rich in a variety of components that can be beneficial for many ailments, like hypertension. But, Allicin, the compound found that is present in garlic and gives it its numerous benefits-doesn't work well when eaten in raw. Consuming garlic in tablet supplement provides the user with excellent results for blood pressure reduction. Be sure to purchase the best quality garlic supplement and use it according to the directions by the manufacturer on its bottle.

Basil

Basil is a popular in the garden that draws beneficial insects. Basil is not only a great addition to your garden, it also goes well with a variety of food items however, it also aids in lowering blood pressure. Research has proven that the extract from basil may reduce blood pressure, although only for a short time. Plant a garden of indoor herbs that contains basil on the kitchen window and just add freshly harvested basil leaves in pasta, salads as well as casseroles and soups. It is not just adding to the taste of the food but will it will also assist in reducing hypertension.

Cinnamon

A delicious and popular food item, it is simple to include in your daily diet and can actually help lower blood pressure. Research has shown that eating cinnamon every day can lower blood pressure for those with diabetes. It is simple to incorporate cinnamon into your daily routine by sprinkled on top of your coffee, oatmeal or cereal. You can also increase the taste of stews, curries and stir-fries by adding a little cinnamon.

Cardamom A spice native to India cardamom is frequently utilized in recipes and dishes that originate from South Asia. A recent study found that patients were given powdered cardamom every day for a period of a few months. The patients experienced a decrease in blood pressure.It's not just powered cardamom which can to lower your blood pressure. It is also possible to include cardamom seeds in baked goods, soups stews, spice rubs, and other dishes.

Celery Seed

The seeds are used to flavor stews and soups, casseroles and other dishes that are savory Celery seed has long been utilized to treat high blood pressure in China. Juicing the entire plant and drinking the juice can also decrease blood pressure. It is believed by experts that it is celery's diuretic qualities that enable the herb to reduce blood pressure.

French Lavender

French lavender is famous for its gorgeous and fragrant flowers. But, this beneficial herb also has a variety of secret properties, including the ability to reduce blood pressure. While many people are apprehensive about an idea to use lavender for a cooking herb, it actually can improve the flavor of your meals. Make use of the leaves the same way as rosemary and keeping the flowers in the oven for baking items.

Cat's Claw

Uncaria Tomentosa is the scientific name for the cat's claw which is a hard climbing vine that is native of Central as well as South America. This plant is covered with hooked thorns that resemble claw of a cat, hence the name. This remedy is extensively used in its home region and has demonstrated promising results to lower blood pressure. It reduces blood pressure through dilation of blood vessels, which allows blood to flow more quickly. Cat's claw also acts in a way of diuretics eliminating sodium and water from your body, thereby reducing hypertension. It is possible to make a decoction by using the fibrous, woody portions of the plant such as the roots or bark. It is similar to a tea that is simmered over longer periods of time. In order to make the cat's claw-decoction, you will require:

1- 2 teaspoons the cat's claw bark that has been dried

1. 1/2- 2 cups of water cold

* Honey or lemon to taste

Then, add the water and dried cat's claw into an unassuming saucepan. Set the saucepan over the stove at a low temperature and cook to a low simmer. Cover the pot and allow it to cook for 30 to 40 minutes. When the time is up remove the dried herb out of the liquid. Add honey or lemon to taste. For the best results, take this mixture every day.

Chapter 19: Corns And Chilblains

Chilblains is a medical condition where exposure to extreme humidity and cold cause damage to tissues. Because of exposure to extreme cold and humidity capillary bed beneath the skin of sufferers are damaged. The skin can get itchy, display many blisters, become red, and suffer from irritation.

The symptoms of Chilblains includeblisters in all affected areas and skin discoloration that it changes from blue to red and, in some instances, lumps of red that appear just beneath the skin. In the most severe cases, ulceration is seen. In some patients the skin is irritated and burning sensations are felt on the affected area.

Corns are painfully thickening of the skin. It is typically caused by excessive pressure. The term used by doctors to describe this skin thickening is Hyperkeratosis. Corns, often referred to as Clavi or Helomas and can be conical or circular shape. The corns are extremely thick, and exhibit the appearance of waxy, translucent or dry appearance.

Corns can cause pain or discomfort while walking

or any other physical exercise.

REMEDIES

A lemon juice drink is well-known remedy that can be rubbed onto corns and then applied to broken Chilblains.

COLDS AND INFLUENZA

Influenza and colds are terms used to describe the effects of viruses. The common cold, also known as "cold" is a respiratory infection that is caused with more than 100 viruses. It's highly infectious and is easily spread through droplets released by sneezing.

The most common symptoms of colds include coughing, sneezing, nasal congestion or runny nasal passage the throat becoming sore and in some instances particularly for children, a mild fever. Patients will typically feel fatigued, experience headaches and occasionally experience pain in their muscles and a lack of appetite.

Influenza commonly known as the "flu," is a viral illness caused by the virus of the Orthomyxoviridae group. It is characterized by symptoms similar as the common cold but it's

usually more severe and may cause severe
respiratory issues.

REMEDIES

Consume plenty of juice from fruit. The juice of
oranges has been considered to be effective for
influenza and colds. The juice of elderberries is
also believed to be one of the best.

The tea of blackcurrants is among the oldest
cures for symptoms of influenza and colds. It is
prepared by adding half a pint boiling water over
one large tablespoonful of blackcurrant jam or
jelly.

Cinnamon tea is another popular solution,
prepared using cinnamon stick boiled in hot water
before filtering the liquid prior to use.

CONSTIPATION

Constipation is a condition in which bowel
movements are more frequent than usual. The
stool gets dry and hard to move. The abdomen
may feel bloated and can cause abdominal
cramps.

Constipation can last for one or two days to a few
weeks. If the frequency of bowel movements is
less than three per week, it is likely that the
person suffering suffers from constipation. An

abdominal bloatedness is extremely painful to live with. It can also hinder appetite because the stomach is apprehensive it's not enough space to hold any food item.

The hard stool is a source of pain during the process of elimination and can easily cause injury to the anal passageway. Additionally, constipation leads to an inability to empty the bowels. This prevents the patient some relief from an empty bowel. If the problem persists abdominal swelling can become a problem and painful. The vomiting can happen when digestion becomes slow. Constipation can be caused by the inability to absorb enough fiber or water and changes in your diet. Whatever the cause, it must be treated quickly to get rid of this lingering discomfort.

REMEDIES

Cracked wheat that has been soaked overnight in water, then boiled for a few hours, is a well-known treatment for constipation.

Olive oil is a mild laxative and is beneficial to add to diets for people suffering from constipation.

Food items to help relieve constipation are Brazil fruit and nuts as well as freshly-picked pineapple, flavored with honey.

DIARRHEA

Diarrhea is the passage of watery stool at least three times per daily. It is believed that the World Health Organization puts diarrhea as the second most common reason for death among children aged less than five. It can last up to two weeks and leave the body totally dehydrated.
It could be caused by an infection bacteria like Salmonella and by food items with excessive roughage, anxiety and in some cases foods that are too spicy.
The biggest risk for people suffering from diarrhea is dehydration due the body's loss of fluid.
If the symptoms persist or are severe, medical advice is recommended.
REMEDIES
Drink plenty of water to fight dehydration.
Fresh raspberries and blackberries are considered to be effective remedies for diarrhea.

ECZEMA

Eczema is a skin disorder that results from inflammation. Sometimes referred to as dermatitis it is a problem that affects a third of all people at least once in their lives. The condition can range from mild or severe, depending on the root cause and treatment. If it is not treated it can worsen which can cause irritation in the skin.

The condition is most commonly present in infants and children but it could be affecting adults as well. The initial symptoms of rashes appear on hands, faces and feet, which can later be spread to other parts of the body.

The most common reasons for eczema are a family history, allergies such as moulds, dust mites and pollens. Wool, among others or wool, low humidity, sweating, dry skin and heat can cause eczema among people. Certain foods like eggs or peanuts, soy and shellfish, as well as fish wheat and nuts may trigger eczema over the face.

The symptoms of eczema are swelling, itching, redness blisters and dry surface, bleeding and leathery skin caused by scratching.

It is crucial to be careful not to scratch the skin because it can result in it breaking, and it could be susceptible to inflammation and infections.

REMEDIES

To ease the irritations of eczema one of the most effective remedies is to apply oil extracted from the kernel of walnuts.

The walnut leaves tree can be used to create an

preparation to wash affected areas. One teaspoon of walnut leaves ought to be simmered in 12 tablespoonfuls of boiling water , and then left to cool prior to use.

FEVER

The symptom of fever is various common ailments. Normal for the body's temperature to fluctuate because of environmental factors like weather, air conditioning, however when the body temperature is far over normal, it is typically referred to as fever however, it's an effect that is a symptom of a different illness.

REMEDIES

Barley is a well-known treatment for fever since they believe it to possess relaxing properties. Since the beginning of time, barley water was an accepted drink for those who are sick.

If using pearl barley in making barley water, it should be cleaned thoroughly. The best results are achieved through washing barley many times with cool water till the liquid is clear.

When barley water is used to treat ailments, it must be potent. This recipe is a great one. 1 pint of barley and 2 1/2 pints water (distilled in the event that it is feasible).

To make barley-water, cook half a pint barley in two and a half pints water for 3 hours or until it is reduced by 2 pints. Strain the mixture and add 4 teaspoons of freshly squeezed lemon juice. Add sweetness to taste using the pure sugar from cane.

The tea of raisin is another popular treatment for fever. To make raisin tea cook half a kilogram washed raisins in two pints water for 4 months or so or until it has decreased down to 1 pint. Sort the liquid through a fine sieve prior to use.

The lemon is also thought to be a good treatment for fever, whether consumed or as drinks made of hot water and lemon juice.

FLATULENCE

Flatulence is a common cause. is eating too much food with an excessive amount of carbohydrates like beans, pulses, the cabbage, lentils and cauliflower. Constipation and air intake can contribute to the condition.

It is characterized by abdominal bloating or discomfort, frequent passage of gas, and vomiting.

REMEDIES

Dietary restrictions on high carbohydrate foods

can reduce the risk of the condition.
For symptoms that are currently present,
common garden thyme is believed by some to
provide relief from flatulence.

Chapter 20: Using Essential Oils For Natural Cures

In addition to food items, there are many other natural resources you can utilize to treat and treat any issue that is ailing you. Essential oils are the direct result of organic materials , and they typically contain the most potent components from the plant.

Here are a few of the most important oils that can be utilized as natural cures

Lavender. The most widely known essential oil contains antiviral and antibacterial properties that can significantly cut down the time required to treat scrapes, stings and bites.

Peppermint. It helps to reduce the symptoms of fever and heat. It can also aid in reducing nausea and motion sickness. Another benefit it can help with is to ease the pain of headaches and migraines.

Eucalyptus. It is often employed as a vaporizer or inhaler, it aids in easing colds and coughs. It cleans and disinfects nasal passages and lungs, helping the patient quickly recover. It also has antibacterial properties, antiviral and antispasmodic.

The oil of Tea Tree. Another powerful antiseptic. It is effective on skin infections caused by fungal organisms, scratches warts insects, cuts and even Dandruff. Most often, it is used as a treatment for acne.

Roman Chamomile. More gentle than tea-tree oil and a more suitable option for skin that is delicate in treating acne scars and acne. It is also used to treat diaper rash as well as eczema.

Jasmine. One of the most costly oils, it is commonly used to ease stress and relax muscles that are tight. It also has been known to boost sexual libido.

Lemongrass. If you are suffering from an infection lemongrass is the best treatment. It is also used to treat infections and is a potent antimicrobial oil, so you can be certain that it will kill any bacteria you apply it.

Chapter 21: Natural Remedies For Hair Loss

What can you do to stop the loss of hair for good? It is a natural process which can be halted and controlled. If you'd like to stop it or grow more strandsof hair, you'll require the assistance of a specialist and undergo medical treatments.

The most one can accomplish is stop it from happening when you can. Learn methods to strengthen and keep your hair healthy and what you can do if you notice indications of hair loss and other hair problems.

Understanding the Issue

In order to determine what to do about the issue it is important to know the reason why you're losing your hair.

1. If you're experiencing hair loss because of a medical issue like thyroid issues bleeding, a lack of vital vitamins in your system, or other health issues, you might need assistance from an expert medical doctor who can solve the issue properly.

Most of the time once the problem is resolved, it

is logical that the effects like hair fall will be cured.

2. You know your self better than anyone else. When your hair starts thin due to your system not getting enough minerals and vitamins, it is time to alter your diet and eat healthy. If it's due to your lifestyle that is unhealthy, begin taking the right steps; make time for exercise, steer clear of the temptations of smoking and drinking and take enough rest.

3. Sometimes, it is enough to handle it in the best way you can. If it is unable to be stopped, try finding ways to hide the issue. If the loss of hair is becoming obvious then you could make use of a hair coloring product to ensure that the contrast with the rest of your hair won't be visible. Look for a product made of natural ingredients that have been proven to be safe and effective. You could also cut your hair shorter or alter the sides on which you split your locks. There are hair products you can utilize to increase the volume of hair and make it appear larger and more full. If you're not satisfied with the outcome You can choose to get hair extensions make sure you select extensions which look like your hair's color and type.

4. It's difficult to watch the lumps of hair falling

off at once, however stressing about it could only make the issue. It is important to know how to manage anxiety. Are there any issues that you should be a concern? If your doctor informs you that you're healthy and that your hair will regenerate, don't get too stressed about it. Focus your thoughts and feelings towards the positive and positive aspect of life. Try breathing and meditation when stress becomes to bear. While doing this, continue taking care of your hair and doing your best take care of it.

1. Eggs. Eggs are a good food source for protein. One method of using this is beating the egg before you apply it to your hair once it's damp. It should be left for 30 minutes, then rinse it off using shampoo and some lukewarm water. This process can be done every week. Another method of using the egg is to extract the egg yolk, and then mix it with your preferred essential oil. Make use of the mixture for massaging your hair from its roots to the tips. Clean it off using the help of lukewarm water. Do not use hot water when washing the egg out of your hair. The egg will be cooked and make it more difficult to remove the egg's particles and odor.

2. Avocado. It is high in vitamin E and is a great

choice as a moisturizer for hair. One method to utilize the fruit would be to smash it in a bowl with a banana, then mix it with one tablespoon of olive oil. Massage your scalp and hair with it, let it sit for 30 minutes before washing it off using Shampoo and water. This could be used to make an hair mask. Mash half this fruit, then mix it in with some spoons of wheat germ oil. Massage your hair with shampoo and apply the mask for hair. Allow it to sit for 20 minutes prior to shampooing your hair a second time and wash it out.

3. Olive oil. It helps give the hair a new life and also strengthens the hair follicles, which helps prevent hair loss. It can be used for massage your scalp and hair. As long as the oil remains warm, apply a gentle massage to your scalp using it, and then leave it for about an hour. You may also cover your head with small piece of cloth or shower cap, and then leave it on top of your head as you rest. Rinse it off using soap and water. It is also possible to use the mixture of honey and olive oil to massage your hair. It should be left for 30 minutes before you wash it off.

Ingram Content Group UK Ltd.
Milton Keynes UK
UKHW020653050623
422889UK00016B/1616